Primary Care
in Urban Disadvantaged
Communities

Edited by

Joe Kai
Professor of Primary Care
University of Nottingham

and

Chris Drinkwater
Professor of Primary Care Development
University of Northumbria at Newcastle

D1438155

Radcliffe Medical Press

Radcliffe Medical Press Ltd
18 Marcham Road
Abingdon
Oxon OX14 1AA
United Kingdom

www.radcliffe-oxford.com
The Radcliffe Medical Press electronic catalogue and online ordering facility.
Direct sales to anywhere in the world.

British Library Cataloguing in Publication Data

A catalogue record for this book is available from the British Library.

ISBN 1 85775 437 9

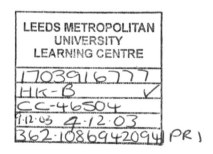
Typeset by Acorn Bookwork, Salisbury, Wiltshire
Printed and bound by TJ International Ltd, Padstow, Cornwall

Contents

About the editors

Joe Kai has been an inner-city GP in Newcastle upon Tyne, then Birmingham and currently practises in central Derby. He is Professor of Primary Care in the Division of Primary Care at the University of Nottingham's Graduate Entry Medical School.

Chris Drinkwater was an inner-city GP in Newcastle upon Tyne for over 20 years and is Company Secretary and Trust Board Member for the West End Health Resource Centre in Benwell. He is Professor of Primary Care Development and Head of the Centre for Primary and Community Learning at the University of Northumbria at Newcastle.

About the contributors

Martin Bennett is Managing Director, Associated Chemists (Wicker) Ltd, Sheffield.

Gillie Bolton writes for patients and clients, and for healthcare, therapeutic and other caring practitioners (Reflective Practice Writing for Professional Development). She is creative writing editor for three medical journals and senior research fellow in Medicine and the Arts at King's College, London.

Philip Crowley has worked in Nicaragua and then Newcastle upon Tyne in community development. Recently trained in public health medicine, he now works in Ireland leading a general practice in a multicultural society initiative and researching child health inequalities with the Institute of Public Health.

Ewan Dick is an Occupational Therapist who joined the Elderly Resource Team in Newcastle at its inception in 1995, subsequently becoming joint co-ordinator of the team while retaining a clinical caseload. He is now Intermediate Care Co-ordinator for Newcastle, leading the Intermediate Care Managed Network.

Mick Down is Director of Pharmaceutical Public Health, Sheffield Health Authority.

Jenny Firth-Cozens has researched, and worked with, stress in doctors and its effects upon patient care. She is Emeritus Professor of Clinical Psychology at Northumbria University and Special Adviser on Modernisation at the London Deanery of Postgraduate Medical Education.

Billy Foreman develops regeneration, health and other partnership initiatives across statutory and voluntary sectors in Birmingham. Previously working in public health for Birmingham Health Authority, he is now Assistant Director of Regeneration and Health at South Birmingham Primary Care Trust.

Debbie Freake is an inner city GP in Newcastle upon Tyne. She has been closely involved in facilitating community partnerships shaping primary care development and commissioning. She is Medical Director of Newcastle Primary Care Trust.

Amanda Howe was a GP at Foxhill Medical Centre in Sheffield, where she worked from 1984–2001. She is now Professor of Primary Care at the University of East Anglia in Norwich where she is a lead member of a new medical school which is in its first academic year.

Jenny Keen is Clinical Director of the Primary Care Clinic for Drug Dependence in Sheffield, a Clinical Research Fellow at the Institute of General Practice and Primary Care, University of Sheffield and Primary Care Regional Lead Clinician, Royal College of General Practitioners.

Shagufta Khan was one of the first local parents to train through Sparkbrook community parents' initiative in Birmingham. She subsequently became an outreach worker for a local Sure Start programme. She now works in community outreach for the regional clinical genetics service.

Siobhan McFeely worked in nursing and general practice for many years before developing outreach sexual health services for young people. Currently she is pursuing a Masters degree in public health; she is a Specialist Development Nurse at North Sheffield Primary Care Trust.

Steve Nash has many years of experience as an occupational therapist and drama therapist in mental health. His service development has included a whole system review of primary care and mental health in North Tyneside. He is now a best practice facilitator with the NHS Modernisation Agency.

Juni Parkhurst qualified as a teacher and used to work with non-school attenders. Also a psychotherapist, she is a freelance trainer, supervisor and coach who specialises in training health professionals in one to one and group work skills. She currently runs a practice, Co-Creative Change, in London.

Stephen Peckham was a health policy academic in Southampton throughout the 1990s. With particular research interests in the relationships between public health, primary care and communities, he is a Reader in Health Policy at Oxford Brookes University.

Claire Pinder joined the Elderly Resource Team in Newcastle in 1995, working as a chiropodist and joint team co-ordinator while managing one of the city day hospitals. She is now a Senior Manager for Rehabilitation and Intermediate Care as part of Newcastle Integrated Older People's Services.

Bethan Plant is a qualified youth worker with longstanding interests and experience working with vulnerable young people. With a Masters degree in public health, she is currently a Senior Health Promotion Manager for children and young people at Sheffield West Primary Care Trust.

Ann Potter was a ward sister, then a health visitor working with families in the disadvantaged West End of Newcastle upon Tyne for many years. She went on to facilitate a community-oriented cardiac rehabilitation programme at the West End Health Resource Centre, and remains active in semi-retirement.

Mary Robson trained as a theatre designer and has worked in the field of arts in health to apply creativity to emotional intelligence and learning, including the Wrekenton Happy Hearts Lanterns Project. She is Project Director of Common Knowledge, the arts in health initiative of Tyne and Wear Health Action Zone.

Jan Smithies has worked in community development and health all her working life. She is a Director of Labyrinth Consultancy and Training Ltd and has recently become a Commissioner to the new Commission for Patient and Public Involvement in Health.

Bhavna Solanki has spent many years working to widen participation and engagement of marginalised communities in health, education and voluntary sectors. She is a programme manager for Sure Start in Birmingham and a board member of Compare, a community charity and business.

Dave Tomson is a general practitioner in North Tyneside with interests in systemic practice and developing whole system service delivery models. He works regionally and nationally to promote innovative education, training and workforce development, particularly in the field of primary care mental health.

Sandra Wathall is a mother and writer with a husband and young son living in Birmingham. She became active in her local Sure Start initiative at its inception and has since been unable to leave.

Acknowledgements

Perhaps this book mirrors its topic. It has had a somewhat tortuous gestation. However, through the persistence and commitment of many people it has, we hope, emerged to capture and celebrate something of value. We are indebted to all of our contributors for joining us in the endeavour. They have taken the time to write, reflect upon and tell their stories despite their many other commitments. We thank them also for graciously accommodating (or at least considering) editorial suggestions and interference. Finally, we thank Kate Billingham as one of the book's originators (before the demands of high office intervened), Paula Moran at Radcliffe for her encouragement and, it goes too often without saying, our families.

Joe Kai
Chris Drinkwater
October 2003

Making surprising things happen: building primary care in urban disadvantaged communities

Chris Drinkwater and Joe Kai

Introduction

All in the developed world face the challenges of regenerating their inner cities and addressing inequalities in health. Primary care does not always seem to feature as part of the solution, although its practitioners deal with the consequences of premature death, abundant mental distress and chronic disease. The demands are such that often stressed and unhappy primary care professionals find themselves working with stressed and unhappy communities. This may be compounded when practitioners find their training has not equipped them for the realities they face as the limitations of the medical model of health are exposed.

This book is written by those working in primary care and community settings. It brings together contributions which examine how primary care is responding to the challenge of urban disadvantage. Through stories and case studies it illustrates the creation and development of new ways of working. They are not necessarily the only 'solutions' but they have been largely successful and appropriate in their local context.

Contributors have been asked to reflect upon what seems to help and what gets in the way. They also note what hasn't worked because we can learn as much, if not more, from our failures as from our successes. The book is intended as an invitation to share learning and discovery with those who have engaged in the struggle to develop and sustain imaginative new approaches.

The strongest common theme is the need to understand and to work within the local context. Surprising things often happen when communities share their views with professionals at the 'front line' and jointly develop responses to local needs. At the same time the challenges that face primary care and urban regeneration at the start of the 21st century must be recognised.

Testing times for primary care and the city

Over the last ten years there has been an explosion in policy making in both primary care and urban regeneration.[1,2] Cynics are inclined to believe that government policy making is a device to retain central control and to keep civil servants and managers busy. A more charitable view is that emerging problems drive policy making. Either way there are major issues about putting policy into practice in the real world of partial evidence, vested interests and resource and capacity constraints.

Primary care and urban regeneration currently confront the same searching question. What is the meaning and purpose of professional practice?[3] And what is the meaning and purpose of the city?[4] Historically the creation of cities and the creation of professional occupations, with medicine as perhaps the most successful profession,[5] have run in parallel over the last 150 years. But both are now challenged. Post-industrial cities are faced with the retreat of people to the suburbs and to rural commuter communities.[6] This undermines the revenue base of the city because of declining income from a per capita poll tax or community charge. It leaves behind an increased concentration of disadvantaged and older people living in public or cheap privately rented accommodation who are financially unable to move.[7] This group are sadly less likely to contribute to the wealth of the city and are more likely to increase costs because of their greater need for services and for subsidised access to public facilities, including transport. As cities become poorer the ability to invest in infrastructure support, such as public transport, declines and, due to the demands of individual commuters in their cars, gridlock results.[8]

In the same way professional practice is also undergoing a paradigm shift. Out goes the autonomous paternalistic professional whose currency is expert knowledge.[9] In comes a more accountable professional whose encounter with the patient becomes a meeting between experts who share knowledge and negotiate solutions. Not surprisingly there is resistance to change. Many professionals are uncomfortable about their reduced autonomy.

Professional practice is seen as less attractive, giving rise to problems with workforce morale, recruitment and retention.[10] This problem is then compounded by the increasing demands made on those who remain. A telling example is the almost tripling of prescription items for anti-depressant drugs from around 9 million in 1991 to 24 million in 2001, with an increased proportion of these prescriptions going to non car owners living in disadvantaged communities.[11]

Structural solutions

In order to address these twin problems, policy makers have focused predominantly on structural solutions. Much of the resource and energy devoted to urban regeneration has focused on demolishing old or no longer desirable buildings and replacing them with new buildings. In the same way, the focus within primary care has been to develop new structures (primary care trusts (PCTs), personal medical service (PMS) pilots to replace the old and apparently redundant.

The problem with a structural approach is that to achieve successful outcomes attention also needs to be paid to processes. The consequence for regeneration initiatives has been that despite significant capital investment many structural initiatives have failed to stop the flow of people from inner city areas. Equally for primary healthcare, structural change has often resulted in decreased rather than increased professional engagement.

Social capital as process

There is some evidence that the need to look at process is beginning to be addressed following the work of Putnam[12] to develop and popularise the concept of 'social capital'. Putnam argues that people and their networks and social relationships can be viewed as a form of (social) capital. This is a resource that needs investment and development in the same way as financial or physical capital.

UK government departments and the Office for National Statistics[13] have now adopted the OECD definition of social capital as the basis for consistent and coherent measurement of its components across the UK. The definition is as follows: 'networks together with shared norms, values and understandings that facilitate co-operation within or among groups'.[14]

Within the UK a survey matrix has now been developed based on work by Blaxter and colleagues.[15] This matrix contains five themes, as follows:

- Participation, social engagement, commitment – involvement in local groups, voluntary organisations, clubs; taking action about a local issue.
- Control, self-efficacy – perceptions of control and influence on community affairs, health, satisfaction with life.
- Perception of community level structures or characteristics – satisfaction with local area; perceptions of local services and local problems.
- Social interaction, social networks, social support – contact with friends, family, neighbours; depth of socialisation networks; perceptions of social support.
- Trust, reciprocity, social cohesion – trust in other people; confidence in institutions; confidence in public services; perceptions of shared values; length of residence in area.

The UK's General Household Survey 2000 included a social capital module for the first time.[16] A study in the United States has demonstrated a strong relationship between poor health and low social capital.[17] Survey data from nearly 170 000 individuals in all fifty states found, as expected, that people who are African American, lack health insurance, are overweight, smoke, have a low income, or lack a college education are at greater risk for illness than more socio-economically advantaged individuals. More importantly, states whose residents were more likely to report poor health were the same states that had low social capital, which was defined as low participation in meetings, low voluntary group membership and low trust of statutory services. Even when the researchers accounted for individual resident's risk factors, the relationship between social capital and individual health remained. Their conclusion was that if one wanted to improve one's health then moving to a high social capital state would do almost as much good as stopping smoking.

Fostering social capital

The need to develop and invest in social capital is now being identified in both health and regeneration policy. Recent publications from the Department of Health include *Shifting the Balance of Power: securing delivery*[18] and *The Expert Patient: A new approach to chronic disease management for the 21st century.*[19] These emphasise the importance of empowerment for patients and the public. *Shifting the Balance of Power* takes this further by stating that 'Staff need to be involved in decisions which affect service delivery. Empowerment comes when staff own the policies and are able to bring about real change'.

In a similar vein, *A New Commitment to Neighbourhood Renewal: national strategy action plan*[20] states that: 'Communities need to be consulted and listened to, and the most effective interventions are often those where communities are actively involved in their design and delivery, and where possible in the driving seat ... But all too often – in the interests of quick results – change has been imposed from above without proper understanding of what the problems are, or there has been no support for communities to get involved. Money goes into neighbourhoods, and leaves them again almost instantly as no funding and no jobs go directly to residents'.

In order to address these issues of empowerment several new proposals have been or are being developed. These include the establishment of a Neighbourhood Renewal Fund and a Community Empowerment Fund targeted at the 88 most deprived local authority districts. For the NHS there are proposals to establish a Staff Involvement Toolkit and to establish Patient Forums (PFs)[21] which will allow local people and communities a greater say in how services are developed and delivered. However welcome these proposals may be in recognising the problem, a number of barriers need to be addressed in order to ensure that the rhetoric matches the reality.

Challenges to increased empowerment of patients, the public and front-line staff

The most significant barriers to addressing this agenda include:

- performance management targets with tight timescales, and perceptions that some targets are more important than others
- trust and respect are essential but fragile commodities, once they are broken they take time to rebuild
- the increasing reliance on quantitative evidence, value for money, evaluation and delivery of outcomes. The risk is that we try to evaluate the impact of empowerment in the same way as we would evaluate a new antibiotic. This ignores the fact that empowerment is a complex, multi-faceted intervention that does not lend itself to traditional positivist research models. Using the wrong models may discredit the whole enterprise. Rather, the focus should be on action research and learning, and on the development of learning organisations.

Trouble with performance management

Both PCTs and local authorities responsible for urban regeneration are subject to an increasingly pervasive performance management system measuring a proliferating number of performance indicators. On the basis of their success or failure in meeting targets they are then given star ratings. These have significant implications for their autonomy and funding, with failing trusts or local authorities being threatened with remedial measures which include the possibility of management teams being replaced.

From the centre, this is clearly seen as a mechanism for exerting control through competition, regulation and supervision. At the front line, however, increasing amounts of time are spent in ritualistic data gathering and gaming, where beating the system becomes more important than improving quality.

The dysfunctional consequences of performance management include concentration on short-term issues to the exclusion of long-term considerations (myopia) and the deliberate manipulation of data by staff – ranging from 'creative' accounting to fraud – so that reported behaviour differs from actual behaviour (misrepresentation).[22] Given known examples of such behaviour, it is perhaps not surprising that some authors have commented that, 'a system that does not trust people begets people that cannot be trusted'.[23] Thus performance measurement, which is in essence motivational or even coercive in nature, may in fact pervert behaviour and engender an adversarial and defensive culture that is detrimental to both quality and to innovation and change.

Trust and respect

One of the consequences of an adversarial and defensive culture is loss of trust and respect. This is clearly reflected in the increasing level of medical litigation, and litigation against local authorities. It is interesting to speculate on whether this is betrayed in the negative stories doctors exchange about patients or patients exchange about doctors.

The reverse side of this is the increased use of reflective practice and approaches such as 'critical friends'[24] and 'patients as teachers'[25] that aim to establish a dialogue of mutual respect between patients and professionals. The outcome of these conflicting approaches is by no means a foregone conclusion. There is certainly evidence to demonstrate that unhappy professionals provide, at best, care without compassion and, at worst, poor or inadequate care.

Richard Sennett has recently argued that we live in a society in which people earn respect when they take care of themselves.[26] Those living in areas of disadvantage who are dependent on welfare lose respect and become subservient victims. This undermines their self-esteem and autonomy and they are less able to make healthy choices for themselves.

This thesis links to work by Wilkinson[27] which has demonstrated that societies with a low income differential between the best and the worst off have better health indicators than societies with large income differentials.

The challenge in the long term then is to reduce income differentials. However, for the health professional in the here and now the challenge is how to build trust and respect with individuals who are often vulnerable and damaged. Increasingly, evidence suggests that this requires time, commitment and continuity. Sennett,[26] for example, quotes a programme for young drug addicts in Paris which presupposes about 18 months to establish an effective network of contacts with the community of drug addicts, and then about five years to wean them individually off drugs.

Developing learning organisations

A learning organisation is an organisation with a memory, which has a clear vision of what it wants to achieve, learns from past mistakes and is pro-active in developing new ways of working.

Nutley and Davies[28] characterise 'learning organisations' as organisations that can configure themselves to maximise, mobilise and retain individual learning. They also describe different levels of learning: single loop learning is about incremental improvements to existing practice; double loop learning occurs when organisations rethink basic goals, norms and paradigms; and meta-learning reflects an organisation's attempts to learn about (and improve) its ability to learn.

They suggest that many organisations never progress beyond single loop learning but that learning organisations attempt to maximise learning capacity by developing skills in double loop learning and meta-learning. This requires organisations to foster open systems thinking which encourages people to explore interconnections across boundaries and for individuals to improve their personal proficiencies within a context of team learning. The organisation also needs to challenge and update implicit assumptions and generalisations so that it can find new ways of doing things, framed by a clear strategic direction and a coherent set of values.

A concrete example of this sort of approach is the West End Health Resource Centre in Newcastle upon Tyne, a Healthy Living Centre that opened in 1996 with a remit to address inequalities in health and to provide support to local people so that they could make their own healthy choices. The centre has developed a model (*see* Figure 1.1), which has equity at the centre and where the other boxes on the diagram relate to important principles about giving local people the opportunity to feel valued within a supportive environment and to have the opportunities for personal and professional development.

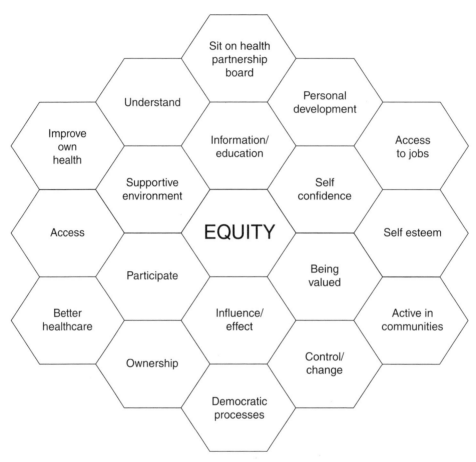

Figure 1.1 West End Health Resource Centre: addressing inequalities in health.

This model could equally well be applied to front-line staff within the NHS, who do not always feel valued or informed. The approach involves the development of complex multi-faceted ways of working. Although it is possible to evaluate separate components, such as the introduction of community-based coronary rehabilitation (*see* Chapter 11), evaluating the whole and demonstrating that the sum is greater than the component parts is a much more difficult enterprise.

Is the time spent on challenging implicit assumptions, reinforcing values and vision, and developing networks worthwhile? Does spending time in this way result in better services which are valued by and meet the needs of users? All of this requires an action research model, which aims at improvement and involvement, involves a cyclic process in which research, action and evaluation are linked and is founded on a research relationship in which those involved are participants in the change process.

Overview

This chapter has described parallels between urban regeneration and current changes within healthcare systems. The major weakness identified is the focus on structures and physical capital at the expense of processes and people and their relationships and networks (social capital). The major opportunity presented is to realise links between social capital, health and empowerment. Yet, there are barriers to empowering patients, the public and front-line staff. These include the dysfunctional effects of an over-reliance on performance management, the erosion of trust and respect between healthcare professionals, patients and the public, and finally the challenge to build learning organisations within a culture that privileges quantitative evidence and delivery of outcomes as 'endpoints' rather than as stages in a process of evolutionary learning.

The above is offered as a context and prelude to this book. The next two chapters provide perceptions of what it is like to work in the inner city by looking at the stories of individuals in a well-established community project and an inner city primary healthcare team. Following these are more theoretical contributions on community-oriented approaches to health, the health of the workforce and community development in primary care (Chapters 4, 5 and 6).

The remaining contributions form the heart of the book (Chapters 7 to 16). They describe a range of projects and practical examples 'at the front line' in different parts of the country. They are about making a difference in responding to the needs of communities and those with heart disease, young families, smokers, younger and older people, mental health, drug misuse and people from diverse ethnic communities.

These accounts illustrate how opportunities to foster people, processes and networks, and thus social capital, empowerment and health, might be negotiated and realised. They offer learning about the very real challenges of doing so and include some reflections on why things sometimes falter. Their common theme is that they challenge implicit assumptions and have developed new ways of working for their local context, which are about valuing communities, service users and front-line staff. Surprising things can then happen.

A concluding chapter considers how such approaches might become mainstreamed and begin to make a real difference. The underlying philosophy is about building trust, respect and social networks not only as a prerequisite to delivering outcomes, but also to enable communities and those working with them to learn and grow.

References

1   Department of Health (2001) *The NHS Plan: A plan for investment. A plan for reform.* Department of Health, London.

2   Cabinet Office (2001) *A New Commitment to Neighbourhood Renewal: National Strategy Action Plan.* Social Exclusion Unit, Cabinet Office, London.

3   Elston AE (1991) The politics of professional power: medicine in a changing health service. In: J Gabe, M Calnan and M Bury (eds) *The Sociology of the Health Service.* Routledge, London.

4   Davis M (2003) *Dead Cities: A natural history.* The New Press, London.

5   Berlant JL (1975) *Profession and Monopoly: A study of medicine in the United States and Great Britain.* University of California Press, California.

6   Muller PO (1981) *Contemporary Suburban America.* Prentice Hall, Englewood Cliffs, NJ.

7   Massey D and Eggers M (1993) The spatial concentration of affluence and poverty during the 1970s. *Urban Aff Q.* **29**: 299–315.

8   Kay JH (1997) *Asphalt Nation: How the automobile took over America and how we can take it back.* Crown, New York.

9   Coulter A (1999) Paternalism or partnership? *BMJ.* **319**: 719–20.

10 Sibbald B, Bojke C and Gravelle H (2003) National survey of job satisfaction and retirement intentions among general practitioners in England. *BMJ.* **326**: 22–4.

11 Society Guardian (2003) Society facts. *Society Guardian.* 5 February: p119. www.society guardian.co.uk

12 Putnam RD (2000) *Bowling Alone: the collapse and revival of American community.* Simon & Schuster, New York.

13 Harper R *The measurement of social capital in the United Kingdom.* www.statistics.gov.uk. (search under 'social capital').

14 Cote S and Healy T (2001) *The Well-being of Nation: the role of human and social capital.* Organisation for Economic Co-operation and Development, Paris.

15 Blaxter M, Poland F and Curran M (2000) *Measuring Social Capital: qualitative study of how older people relate social capital to health.* Final Report to the Health Development Agency, London.

16 Coulthard M, Walker W and Morgan A (2002) *People's Perceptions of Their Neighbourhood and Community Involvement: results from the social capital module of the General Household Survey 2000.* The Stationery Office, London.

17 Kawachi I, Kennedy BP and Glass R (1999) Social capital and self-rated health: a contextual analysis. *Am J Pub Health.* **89**: 1187–93.

18 Department of Health (2001) *Shifting the Balance of Power: securing delivery*. Department of Health, London.

19 Department of Health (2001) *The Expert Patient: a new approach to chronic disease management for the 21st century*. Department of Health, London.

20 Cabinet Office (2001) *A New Commitment to Neighbourhood Renewal: national strategy action plan*. Social Exclusion Unit, Cabinet Office, London.

21 Department of Health (2001) *Involving Patients and the Public in Healthcare: A discussion document*. Department of Health, London.

22 Goddard M and Smith PC (2001) Performance measurement in the New NHS. *Health Policy Matters*. Issue 3: January. University of York, York.

23 Davies HTO and Lampel J (1998) Trust in performance indicators? *Qual Health Care*. 7: 159–62.

24 Fisher B and Gilbert D (2001) Patient involvement and clinical effectiveness. In: F Brooks and S Gillams (eds) *New Beginnings*. Kings Fund, London.

25 Greco M and Carter M (2001) *Establishing Critical Friends Groups in General Practice*. Report to the North and East Devon Health Authority, Exeter and North Devon NHS Research and Development Support Unit.

26 Sennett R (2003) *Respect: the formation of character in an age of inequality*. Allen Lane; Penguin Press, London.

27 Wilkinson RG (1996) *Unhealthy Societies: The afflictions of inequality*. Routledge, New York.

28 Nutley SM and Davies HTO (2001) Developing organisational learning in the NHS. *Med Educ*. 35(1):35–42.

CHAPTER 2

Riverside Community Health Project: workers' stories

Gillie Bolton

'It's called a health project ... but they do a bit of all sorts there' [1]

The sun is shining over the hill on the other side of the valley, showing up the houses in serried ranks, interleaved with bright, green, early spring fields after the deluge of rain. But the wind is biting. People scurry up and down the steep hill with heavy shopping bags, or into the Edwardian stone library, clutching children's hands. This library is at the intersection of four dense housing areas in the west end of Newcastle upon Tyne. Some are so unpopular that the houses are being mown down and replaced by industrial units, or just scarred ground – creating even more stress in an already stressed area.

The basement of this library is The Riverside Community Health Project. A bright, welcoming place full of children, children's artwork and animated people. In the words of the Bangladeshi family and community support worker, Nazrul Islam, Riverside is 'a locally managed, voluntary sector organisation, which works with many disadvantaged communities in our neighbourhood, and addresses inequities in health'. Riverside's primary aim is empowerment of local people. The main method chosen to achieve this is a multi-pronged approach linking social action in the local neighbourhood with work on policy issues, research on health matters, influence on professional practice, and inter-agency collaboration. Its formal independence from statutory services and agencies is seen as a strength, enabling the community workers to act in an advocacy role for communities and to work in partnership with local people.

The main focus of the project's work is the general field of health and well being. However, its commitment to a social model of health means that its work inevitably extends into areas of concern, such as housing policy and income maintenance.[1]

But this basement was not always so, as Marge Craig depicts:

'A huge cave of a space – dark, filthy, very damp with a little stream running across the dirt floor, loads of junk from the last eighty years. Most unpromising. But we thought it was great. We felt so much excitement about all the things we would be able to do in our own space. Especially compared to where we were before – up three flights to a spare classroom in the school – mums struggling with buggies and trying to talk over the noise of little ones playing.'

Reflective practice writing

This chapter draws on work I was doing with people at Riverside – reflective practice writing for professional development. This can enable practitioners to identify and reflect upon areas of their experience which need enquiring into in whatever way is appropriate.[2,3] The process involves focused creative writing exercises and effectively facilitated educational small group work. The former harnesses the power of explorative and expressive writing to offer immediate and focused contact with personally vital issues. It is qualitatively different from a talk-based process. Sharing such writings to support change and development is undertaken in a carefully facilitated, trusting, confidential forum. I tell more about this process at Riverside later on in the chapter. But first some of what was written.

Riverside told by workers

Carol Willis wrote of her feelings about the bulldozing of so many houses in their area, and how this reminded her of the West end in the past as she remembers it:

'When the plans for demolishing houses in the west end broke, it reminded me that this is all happening again, like when T Dan Smith was around in the mid-60s – but then it all sort of happened, without consultation – slum clearance. I remember one woman who owned her own house, she stuck out for getting the right price for it and they started demolishing her terrace at both ends and she hung out a white flag to surrender. The difference between then and now is that she wouldn't have been in negative equity on her mortgage, she wouldn't have had to go on paying a mortgage for the rubble left behind.

They demolished everything around us except South View Terrace, this little row of houses, and we eventually moved into a house there – a huge, solid terrace house with bay windows and a lovely staircase – which was pulled down later.

All our friends and neighbours were disappearing, the community was lost, leaving us isolated, putting up with the dust and everything happening around us. Just like people are now. Now when I see that empty piece of land I think what a shame, what once was a solid house is now a car park space for the factory.

Lost all of the shops. In fact the butcher who had a shop in Scotswood used to deliver the meat in his little van to that row of houses. There wasn't even a corner shop anywhere except for MacDonald Road. Quite often, younger people would get bits of shopping for older people who couldn't make it up the hill.

At least people have a chance to have a say this time round, whether that'll make a difference, but that's different from last time. I think about the little bit left on Buddle Road which is in the same situation – totally isolated. But we were able to move into a new house on the Guinness Trust estate which was being built, but the people who'd been shifted earlier did not have the choice to stay in the area.

I think about the people who lived in the little Tyneside flats in the streets running down the hill, with no inside toilets, and maybe it was a 'nice new house' so there was a lot of mixed feelings. It's different now – people have made their homes and they don't want to have the plans imposed on them.'

Marge Craig continues with what she feels the Riverside Centre is all about:

'Independence is the key to set all women free – it's so true, and I think it's what our work is all about – relationships, and the economic independence and confidence for women who are at **the most vulnerable stage of their adult life** – when they've got babies and children who are dependent on them, when they're exhausted, anxious, dependent on others' goodwill, fed up, exhausted, exhausted, exhausted. See them come here for solace, to recharge their batteries, to tell us how bad it is, and, **also**, to have a laugh, take a break, do something for themselves, put their heads above the parapet and **know** there is a life out there.

Yesterday when Joanne set off home in the pouring rain with baby and toddler, she said 'we're better off than people in Ethiopia where they've not had rain for three years'. Made my day. 'Cos I worry about the insularity, cut-off-ness from the wider world of some women, understandably when overwhelmed by day-to-day concerns – crying babies, exhaustion, exhaustion . . . .'

And who are these women? Nazrul Islam takes up the story:

'Rahima is a Bangladeshi woman. She has been brought up in a village in Bangladesh with lots of family and friends. A small river passes near her village, with a rice field nearby covered with green rice crops. Green trees surround all houses in the village. Every household has a pond where fishes are kept. During the summer season it's almost always hot with long summery days, people are outside, with all doors and windows open. Everybody gets together and socialises in a cheerful mood. Mothers get plenty of help with childcare from family and friends. From this hot summery, cheerful environment, Rahima emigrated to England where she had plenty of hope and wished for a good life.

Once Rahima came to England she lost all family contact. She found it very difficult to adapt to a different culture and environment. She is indoors constantly, feeling isolated as she does not speak any English and is unfamiliar with the local area and people. She does not have anyone to talk to properly as her husband works 70 hours a week in a Bangladeshi restaurant, and she does not have much support with her two small children.

Rahima tends to worry a lot. Her health is deteriorating and she tends to feel depressed most of the time, and seems to be getting symptoms of mental health problems. Her hopes and dreams of living a happy life in England have now become a nightmare.'

And another family, from Carol Willis:

'K, M and their 3-year-old son, D, are refugees from Yugoslavia. Much of my work was spent settling them and other families into our community. I thought that at least they were safe and comfortable here in their new home and would be able to build a new life. I did everything in the way of practical support and friendship and, even though there was a language barrier, we managed.

K became pregnant with twins, which brought happiness to their lives, but early in the pregnancy one of the babies died. After the premature birth of the second twin the hospital staff asked me to come with her to the special baby unit while they explained that her baby may not live that night.

This was the first time I had been into a special care baby unit; I remember very clearly seeing this tiny black, almost doll-like life in the incubator and finding it so hard not to cry. Feeling very helpless I left when her husband arrived, leaving them to share their grief in privacy.

I helped K choose flowers for their funeral and attended the service with other workers and friends. It was K and M's hope that after a few months they would be able to try for another baby. But within a short time M was diagnosed with angina which was hereditary. Over the coming weeks M's health deteriorated, and he was further diagnosed with liver cancer, which was to take his life very quickly. M's mother, also in poor health, came to join the family.

While M was in hospital I remember one of the worst rain storms we had had in a long time. In desperation K rang me at home in the evening as the water level had risen to the doorstep of her front door. I rang the 24-hour emergency service provided by the housing association, only to be told that they can't help unless the water is actually flooding into the house. I rang K and explained the situation to her bearing in mind her limited amount of English and my lack of her own language. I told her to ring me back, no matter what time, if the water started to come into the house. I looked out of the window up at the sky, and thought 'dear God please let the rain stop, poor K has enough happening to her without this'. Next morning I went to see her and the water had reached to within an inch of flooding into the house. Was it by the hand of God, perhaps realistically a meteorological explanation. At least now the housing association are investigating why the drainage system is unable to cope.

It was a sunny day in August when I went with a refugee worker and K and D, to visit M in the hospice. I watched as D skipped though the gardens unaware of his daddy's fate. M's mother developed a secondary cancer and died Friday 22 October aged 49, M died 30 October aged 29 years.

K is now building a new life for her and D. Her stay in England has been extended for four years, and she has just completed the first part of a computer course. Her English has improved greatly, and her confidence is growing. A Kosovan family, her only friends, have just moved into the house next door.'

Making a difference

The staff at Riverside Centre, many of whom live in the area, help Rahima, K and D and many others in so many ways. Kath Gains describes the beginnings of the holiday club:

'Many volunteers set the wheels in motion. A holiday association was set up, and we invited families from the west end to come along. A small weekly fee was set for each family and the fundraising started with vigour and enthusiasm. The centre was a hive of activity with social events, raffles, car-boot sales and funding applications made. Nobody minded helping, after all they were going on holiday. How exciting!

Could we possibly pull this off? Would it all go smoothly? Of course it would. The twenty-first of August arrived and it was time to set off for Berwick Holiday Site. Thirty-seven families, children excited, mothers frantic, "have we got everything? I just know I've left something behind." And we're off. We arrived on coaches, in cars and vans, the cries from the children "wow this is excellent", "look at the sea, the amusements", "Mum, Dad, can I have some money please?" "We've just got here, can't you wait?" The week came and went, and everyone had a fabulous time. At the end of the week it was very emotional. The gratitude from everybody, "thanks for an excellent time", "thanks for making this happen for us", "we wouldn't have had a holiday otherwise". What a feeling.'

And Mandy Whitfield's description of an event:

'I really enjoyed being a clown along with one of our crèche workers at an event we held at South Benwell School a few years ago. I liked being a clown because the kids were coming up to me and you could see how happy they were, laughing at my big shoes and red nose. I've just remembered my legs were killing me at the end of the day though, having to lift them so high to walk in the shoes.'

The holiday and the clown event are high points. Life and work at Riverside and its environs are often very different. Anne Bonner describes her feelings occasioned by meetings in which many different people with different interests are deciding how they should proceed with projects such as the holiday club. At the Riverside Project decisions are made by the whole group involved, rather than just the staff, a correct but notoriously tricky way to conduct matters.

'There is no real dividing line between the life of the community and the life of the Riverside Project, our work is about everyday lived experience. And, this is not a nine-to-five job. We go home and keep seeing people. They are so helpless and I can't shut my door. And the staff feel they celebrate their real contact with people. Even if it is difficult, it's rewarding.'

Although many staff live in the area, and are therefore members of the community, this doesn't necessarily give them insight into the best way for them to be working at Riverside, 'we realise we are a very small part of the people's lives. There is so much we don't know, so many ways we don't know what's right and what's wrong for them.' And it's not only the moral, ethical and social dilemmas which make such work difficult, but also personal ones.

Derek Snaith focused upon feedback he received which gave him 'the realisation that I am doing something right within my work', and how that felt:

'She said that I was a key worker because I had helped start a social club for adults with learning difficulties in the area. What I had never realised in all my time here at Riverside was that my work was making a difference to people. I could tell from the passion in her voice that this initiative "The Millennium Club" is something she and others have been looking for for years. And I still am shocked when positive feedback comes from those involved in helping to run the sessions and those who come along to enjoy it.

This simple statement, and the subsequent realisation of the impact of my work, has helped me in my mind to be more confident in my own abilities and my own views. I think I will be able to be myself more at work and be more assertive when it comes to dealing with people and groups who are there purely for self-interest or generally negative reasons.

Because I now know that I have made a difference to people who are in need of supporters to do things for them and alongside them. It means I can stick my neck out and say more of what I think clearly, rather than a watered down mish-mash that is often not understood.'

Writing the stories

These accounts from Riverside were created during a morning's workshop run to support staff in reflecting together upon the experience of their work. It offered them space away from the everyday busy-ness of running the Project: 'we *never* normally *talk* to each other like this about what we *feel* and *think* about our work and the lives of the people with whom we work.'

I have been doing this kind of work for many years, encouraging groups of primary care staff (medical, nursing, support, admin, therapeutic, as well as social workers, educators and other groupings) to reflect effectively by writing stories or poems about their work and discussing with each other whatever needs discussing arising from the writings.[2–5] It is not ideal to work with a group for only a few sessions as we did at Riverside. With several sessions a group can develop trust and confidence in the process, and be more courageous in what they are willing and able to share. But the close and trusting working relationships at Riverside enabled us to get a very long way in a very short time. In more sessions staff can begin to move outwards in their reflection, write in the voice of a client or patient for example, try out how events might have been different had they been more assertive, or if the genders of the main people involved had been different. But what we had was good.

Children thumped about in the library overhead as we wrote and talked. And more children laughed, cried, played in the other rooms of the Riverside Project. The everyday business of the life of the Riverside Project ebbed and flowed around us, leaving a clear pool for us in the middle – for us to reflect within.

Space for reflection

The heart of the reflective workshop was writing. I asked each to write a story about a vital event in their working lives. Pens and pencils scribbled like mad. We then re-read our writing silently to ourselves – to acquaint ourselves with what we had written at such speed. And then we read the pieces to each other, with space for as much discussion as was needed on the issues raised by the writings of the staff involved. It was a warm and close occasion – a space they said they never normally take – a couple of hours to allow themselves to reflect deeply and silently on their own in the writing, and then in thoughtful discussion with each other.

Many of the group shared feelings, hopes and anxieties, which surprised the rest of the group; it isn't always easy in the busy turmoil of the day-to-day working of a place like this to share hesitancies. For example, they were amazed that Derek needed that feedback to assure him of the value of his work. They were able to reinforce the positive feedback he had already been offered, in good measure. And one other staff member wrote about the way a negative encounter had knocked her confidence. Once more the group were very surprised – not realising she was not as confident as she seemed. They were able to offer real support.

The discussion was interspersed with thoughtful silences, laughter, anxieties and tensions at difficult memories, but always a warm supportive sharing, and a keen interest and care for the people in their community. One said they were 'stopping the speed of life to take time to reflect upon important things, and talk properly to each other'.

Coda

At Riverside they also sing. As I left, the table and chairs we'd used were pushed back and the big room filled with a circle of women and babies, and the sound of glad voices. As one commented, 'I thoroughly enjoyed the singing – very friendly and lovely to be here and what a way to end the week – on a high note!'

Staff and community residents sang together. But at Riverside the distinction is difficult to make. Many staff are also resident in the area, and all are located here in their hearts. Similarly, the voices you have read in the above writings are from staff, but they also poignantly reflect local people's voices.

The staff group commented of their community, 'we feel like an island, at times, in a storm-tossed sea of government statistics'. The writings created by these seven people offer a window into this island, into this vibrant health project in an inner urban community.

Acknowledgements

I would like to thank Anne Bonner, Marge Craig, Kath Gains, Nazrul Islam, Derek Snaith, Mandy Whitfield and Carol Willis for most stimulating reflective writing sessions, and for their generous permission to quote from their writings and what they said (all names are fictionalised). Their voices shine through in this chapter.

References

1   Green J (1996) *Summary report of an evaluation of the Riverside Community Health Project*. Social Welfare Research Unit, University of Northumbria in Newcastle.

2   Bolton G (2001) *Reflective Practice Writing for Professional Development*. Sage, London.

3   Bolton G (1999) Stories at work: reflective writing for practitioners. *Lancet*. **354**: 243–5.

4   Winter R, Buck A and Sobiechowska P (1999) *Professional experience and the Investigative Imagination: the art of reflective writing*. Routledge, London.

5   Bleakley A (2000) Writing with invisible ink: narrative, confessionalism and reflective practice. *Reflective Practice*. 1:1 11–24.

CHAPTER 3

Foxhill – an out of the ordinary story of inner city teamwork

Co-ordinated by Amanda Howe, for all members of Foxhill primary care team

Introduction

In this chapter, through writing and reflection, we will try to describe not only what we feel makes us a good team, but also how we have arrived at, and try to maintain, this happy point. The writing below has two parts – a historical 'story', and team contributions on the here and now. We have used literature from others to support our views, but have avoided an academic analysis. The key factors underpinning successful teamwork are well known.[1] Our story is personal, partial, capturing the moment. We think we are special and different. But we are not alone, not so extraordinary in our shared commitment to work in Foxhill. We know that others choose to work in areas of burgeoning unemployment, vandalism and drug addiction, soiled streets and endless dogged courage. We hope our work will help encourage others to work in inner cities, and to thrive within the challenges they represent.

Foxhill

First a little about Foxhill. A little known working class area of northwest Sheffield, boundaried by the moors and spaces that famously edge the city. It is bypassed by fans heading to the infamous Hillsborough football ground, and by the traffic that streams along a dangerous dual carriageway which dissects Foxhill from other equally deprived communities. On that road, at a junction that manages to sustain a road accident at least once a week, sits a much extended family house with a sign offering welcome to new patients. This is Foxhill Medical Centre.

Foxhill has had a neighbourhood practice since the post-war era, when a single-handed doctor set up his home and business there. Twenty years ago, when his children's nanny doubled as receptionist and doorkeeper, he took on an assistant. This doctor, a motorbike fanatic, was often mistaken for a tradesman in his early days at the practice – much to the subsequent embarrassment of patients involved in our particular urban myths. He, a practice nurse, and the practice counsellor are the only staff that remain from the heady days of the early eighties, when the NHS went unquestioned in its excellence as a public service. The shift from small business to health centre was untramelled by managerial direction, and there was space for innovation in practice. The stories one could tell about Foxhill therefore involve many eras, many people, and a multiplicity of teams.

Amanda's story: *tips for recruiting to the inner city*

Start young

I first came to Foxhill as a GP registrar in training at the mature and blooded age of 27. I had known staff there in the primary healthcare scene through my previous two years on the vocational training scheme. Perhaps this is a first tip – the role model function of the established practitioner, which will draw like minds towards it from a younger cohort. I could see that good committed staff worked at Foxhill and were trying to change things – for the people of the area rather than themselves. So, if you want to get people to work in the inner city, ensure exposure to those who have already engaged.

As I started to work there, doing on call overnight, I found the partners caring and concerned. They were also desperate for my help in the very high workload area, so I felt needed, encouraged. I was not thought crazy by my own personal circle, but some of my peers expressed surprise. Already we had divided into those who preferred the inner city and those who were headed for higher pay and leafy suburbs. A second tip – political and attitudinal factors seem well defined by the graduate stage, so shaping the cultural expectations of young doctors needs to start early.[2]

The attractions of patients

I subsequently became a locum in the practice. Tip three – allow potential staff to sample, to work without long-term commitment, to be nurtured into showing them that they can cope – and enjoy it! After six months, I was happy to accept a partnership: partly because of the patients.

A committed GP will enjoy the majority of patient contact because it is a necessary skill of their speciality. For me there was something special about the patients of our urban and deprived community. They were different from me, invoked no stifling propriety or parental resonances. They bore living conditions with incredible ingenuity and fortitude that I had never learned to tolerate. On the whole, they accepted the inevitable sufferings of illness and death with an openness and responsibility that I had not experienced elsewhere. As a young person still unaccustomed to the human condition I learned much from them as I attempted to respond to their needs. Tip number four – do not stereotype the difficulties of inner city work to the extent where they outweigh the pleasures, because this would not reflect our experience!

Coping strategies

Nevertheless, as a member of staff there were some specific problems worth reflecting upon. The workload was horrendous, the building archaic, the night life a little dodgy (fierce dogs on the loose, car vandalism, the occasional snatched bag), and some of the patients a danger both to themselves and to others. How does a good team cope? Our mechanisms were:

- a convention of telling and listening (even if it means home at 8.00 pm instead of 7.30 pm)
- generous leave conditions (even if a low salary)
- taking the load from whoever is going under, if possible
- a reciprocity that relies on knowing that others in the team respect and do not judge you.

Having said that, we were unkind to ourselves. Today's GPs may never know the strain of a whole weekend on call, when you neither relied on partners nor a co-operative to bail you out, however busy. Another principle learned – there is a point beyond which working in the inner city becomes intolerable. All practices should ensure that staff can 'opt out' at the point just before they become unsafe, or when the environment becomes unsafe for them.

Team ebbs and flows

Over the years, as the practice modernised, we lost three administrative staff who had come from and served the community for many years. The need for change, coupled with altered expectations of each team member, led to bad feeling and eventually a parting of the ways, which was both painful and costly. We also lost a colleague who combined a devotion to patients with a deep sense of duty and a lack of personal boundaries. This was dangerous in a practice like ours, where the need is endless. Others left for less traumatic reasons.

More positively, and unlike many others, there was never a split in the GP partnership itself, and all previous partners still keep in contact. The average length of service in the partnership is low, but this is because of the culture of accepting change. We were a salaried pilot long before the government invented these and our 'no buy in or out' clause has allowed partners to take up other lives and posts with goodwill rather than bitterness.

Sustaining it through innovation

We struggled with the management role of the GP, trying various approaches that accorded more with our beliefs about teamwork than the needs for performance, and have now settled into a model that seems to work (see below). Also, we always tried to embrace others into the team. We have greatly benefited from the common endeavour of community nursing and health visitor colleagues, who have worked beyond the conventional boundaries to deliver important services in a way that the more erratic and damaged patients can handle.

Another tip for viability – innovation. We have often been pulled together by new projects when the daily grind has kept us fragmented, rushing into our separate rooms and cars, undergoing our own unique pattern of patient care. Whether it be a whole food shop, a drug addiction service, herbalism or family therapy, creative staff who would otherwise have burnt out in the commonplace have made time to deliver new opportunities, and in the process have learned from, and extended the skills of, many other team members. We have researched together, taught and trained others on a continuous basis, and contributed to service development initiatives for the city as a whole. And we have played together – nights out, seaside outings with the community groups, creative writing workshops, dancing. Even our staff development days are overtaken by humour and games.

Foxhill was a large part of my adult life – 18 years. I have tried to show what drew me there, what made it survivable in spite of many traumas, and why I worked there until 2001. I am, and have always been, grateful for the privilege.

Ian's bad day

A typical surgery at Foxhill is always demanding, as described by Ian Nerurkar in this excerpt from his account called *Bad Day*:

'So, here we go ...

1 Lecturer stressed out by work but declining suggestions of help.
2 Two problems in 8 minutes (with missing notes – because the first of the problems was already being dealt with in the 'system'). The second is oedema.
3 Three problems in 8 minutes: pill check, lump in neck, tired all the time and stress (alcoholic partner, son with behavioural problems, debt complaints).
4 Boyfriend problems / stress ... review (why does she want to come back so soon?).
5 Two easy minor complaints (thank God for a break).
6 Long standing tension headaches, CT scan at last GP was normal, mother died of brain tumour. Doesn't like any discussion of non-organic factors.
7 Sciatica (easy though painful – but I feel bad not reviewing his previous history of epilepsy fully today, as he doesn't often come in).
8 Miscarriage last week, needs someone to talk to. Unsupportive partner (well known to me), previous husband violent, sexually abused as a child, raped and stalked by a drug addict who won't be prosecuted because he is a police informer.
9 Parents of adolescent children with drug and truancy problems (not to mention the renal failure, rejected transplant and home dialysis ...) accompanied by a friendly but 'time consuming' Educational Welfare Officer allocated to one of the sons.

And so on ...

I'm finished. At last. Exhausted. Tension headache and bellyache. And then, there is a visit after surgery, 'can't come down...'. My fuse goes – BAAANGG!!, I blow immediately, feel better and worse for it. I apologise to the receptionists, and explain. They leave. How do they feel now? Will they come back tomorrow? What do they / will they think of me?'

What makes a good team?

So, how do we help each other to deal with these situations, daily, year after year? Many see the other members of the team as their coping resource in the face of severe demand. But what makes us a good team? Personal comments for this chapter did not come in 'book speak' but there were recurrent themes raised by staff at Foxhill which echo those of research studies. Take for example, the following observations on good teamwork, from Matt James, who was a GP registrar training at Foxhill for six months.

- 'All members of the team are valued and respected so there is an easy openness which seems to stop tension.
- Regular meetings and a relaxed atmosphere help this, also openness that extends to thinking as well as people.'

These resonate with the recommendations from research that effective teamwork needs to offer regular participation to all members, and to make all feel important to the fate of the group.[3]

Others described the strongly held group identity which allows us to appraise and, if necessary, oppose those forces which conflict with our own deeply held values. Although such attitudes may appear confrontational, they can form useful 'defence mechanisms' when faced with inappropriate demands. Tom Heller captured this in his poem below.

Visitors to Foxhill

Tom Heller

When people from outside come to visit us
To our team meetings
We eat them, we really do

They come when they want us to do more things
More forms to fill
More hoops to jump

So we eat them
With sauce
With panache, with style

We might listen for a while
Ask a few questions, polite like

Then kebab them
Roast them, hoist them on their own acronyms

We don't mean to do it
Honest
But we just can't resist

What do they know
Of life on the estate
Of being abused?

What do they know
Of being poor
Or scrabbling for air?

And what do they know of us who work there?
Who stay alongside those in trouble
Who hold their hands in the night
And listen to their first and last breaths
And the wheezing and puffing in between

And the stories they tell us
Of hopes dashed
Lives destroyed
Of bodies deformed

So don't come to us with your schemes for change
For 'reforms' not thought through
For payments withheld
For targets unmet

We'll eat you
We really will.

Promoting involvement

Some of the philosophy that has driven Foxhill parallels the latest work on good practice in empowerment.[4] Just as we try to promote active patient involvement in self-care, we also promote this for staff – 'full involvement and control' being reflected in our explicit meeting structure which allows all staff groups some involvement in management.

Weekly meetings	Monthly meetings
General practitioners	(week on week rotation)
Management group	Practice meeting
(practice manager,	All clinical staff
GP executive partner,	Case discussions
senior receptionist, and	Worker group discussion
clinical representative)	

This has not always been easy or indeed popular. Staff unused to participating in flat hierarchy organisations took many years to trust or relate to this structure. At the same time, there are always means by which the most representative structures can be sidelined if a powerful individual or group has other intentions. However, this structure allows any subversion of the decision-making structures to be openly and repeatedly corrected.

Teaching and service development

Another aspect that has pulled us together is training and teaching. A study involving some of our staff showed that primary care teams experienced the challenge of delivering community based medical education placements for undergraduates as enhancing team work, presumably as would any coordinated activity for a new shared task.[5] Certainly such activities are required to enable students to experience the reality of teamwork for clinical practice, and become good team players.

And then there are new projects, such as our Healthy Living Centre. Visioning new undertakings, embracing new possibilities, is another characteristic of the good team, and allows us to extend our own roles in previously unappreciated ways.

Team building at Foxhill

Tom Heller

How do we know what we are building?
We haven't built it yet.

But we are building something together
It's got a silhouette
Like the ribs of a shipyard against the sky
When you get nearer,
You can hear it, each person working
Constructing something with many shapes
Shapes and images keep it going

They fit together; an organism, a living thing
Taking on the characteristics of the constructing team
And it's moving forwards, rolling, rumbling
It may be gathering speed
Developing, metamorphosing, incorporating
New shapes you might not recognise.

Conclusion

We can only make some recommendations:

- find others who are driven by the same values as you
- create structures that reflect those values
- ensure flexible and supportive working conditions (to compensate for the hard work, the drain of dealing with deprivation, and the possibility that people will need to leave or change)
- choose those who are motivated by a wish to work in this type of practice with these kind of clients
- refuse those who you suspect are 'unboundaried' or have poor survival mechanisms.

And finally, consider the virtues of the Foxhill Ten Commandments (with thanks to Helen Drucquer):

1 All chocolate to be shared.
2 All pompous bubbles to be pricked.
3 All tears, fears and cares to be respected.
4 All heartsink patients to be seen as beautiful.
5 If heart does sink, know that you have met another in truth.
6 Laugh – but not all the way to the bank.
7 All strengths to be known from inside, not judged from without.
8 Bereavements, births and blessings to be seen as life events that need time, love (and a continuing salary).
9 All protocols to be seen as necessary rules that can, and sometimes must, be broken.
10 The child within to be allowed to play.

References

1   West M (1994) *Effective Teamwork.* BPS Books (British Psychological Society), Leicester.

2   Habbick BF and Leeder SR (1996) Orienting medical education to community need: a review. *Med Educ.* **30**: 163–71.

3   West M and Poulton B (1997) Primary care teams: in a league of their own. In: P Pearson and J Spencer (eds) *Promoting Teamwork in Primary Care.* Arnold, London.

4   Sturt J (1998) Implementing theory into health promotion practice: an empowering approach. In: S Kendall (ed) *Health and Empowerment: research and practice.* Arnold, London.

5   Howe A (2000) Teaching in practice – a qualitative factor analysis of community based teaching. *Med Educ.* **34** (9): 762–8.

Community oriented approaches to health: reconciling individual and community needs

Stephen Peckham

Introduction

Many factors may contribute to an individual's health or to the health of a 'community'. However, the health of a community is not simply the sum of individual health within a given community. Health is also derived from being part of a community, from the extra benefit or well being which the community provides. Public health activities often focus on geographical communities such as neighbourhoods. Yet, communities are also made up of people who share similar experiences in health (such as people with mental health problems or diabetes) or similar characteristics such as a shared cultural or ethnic background.

A distinction might be drawn between the delivery of medical care to individuals and the pursuance of public health that focuses on the whole community. However, there are other dichotomies. Firstly, between the medical model of health which emphasises biological factors, and the more holistic social model of health which acknowledges physical and social as well as biological factors. Secondly, the tension between lay and expert perspectives about health provision and outcomes and who creates health.

This chapter explores these relationships and how perceived tensions can be overcome. It draws upon recent research and the experiences of local communities to offer an account of how individual and community health can be reconciled by providing an overview of community oriented approaches to health.

Healthy individuals, communities and social capital

Both community based and individual approaches to public health are seen as playing complementary roles.[1,2] Traditionally, the health of a community has been measured by aggregating the health of individuals (e.g. by combining measures of morbidity and mortality). However, recent research suggests health also depends on the health of a community, as a *community*.[3] As the examples later in this chapter may demonstrate, the development of a healthy community is in itself beneficial to individual health. This concept of so-called 'social capital' is not new. Community involvement in health was central to the development of the Peckham Health Centre in the 1930s, but is once again informing public health.[1,4]

Social capital is based on the idea of social cohesion, which is the measure of community relations. The more socially cohesive a community the more networks, community activity and strong inter-relationships exist.[3] Social capital has been described as the '... features of social life – networks, norms, and trust – that enable participants to act together more effectively to pursue shared objectives ... To the extent that the norms, networks, and trust link substantial sectors of the community and span underlying social cleavages...'[5]

Notions of community

The notion of 'community' has been debated for many years. It can be used to describe local populations and a focus for local service delivery. This includes locality approaches to healthcare such as primary care services[6] and healthy living centres.[1] There is a renewed focus on health inequalities within communities reflecting concerns raised in the 1980s in the *Black Report* and the *Health Divide*.[7]

In these circumstances, communities are seen as geographical areas rather than other forms of community such as patient and local voluntary and community groups. The inter-relationship between such 'communities of interest' and geographical area is often overlooked. In reality communities represent a complex network of formal and informal relationships (see Table 4.1).

Table 4.1: Individual and community relationships

Who	Act as	How	Who with	Comments
Individuals	Patients, health providers	Self care, shared care, user involvement, complaints	Themselves, health professionals, other users	Predominantly a medical model operating Example: individual practitioner consultations
Families	Patients, health providers, carers/parents, supporters, advocates		Themselves, health professionals	Represents a family orientation usually within primary medical care Example: UK general practice
Informal networks	Supporters, health providers	Friend and kinship networks, self help groups	Themselves, health professionals	May work collaboratively with specific health professionals but main emphasis is on mutual support. Example: Carers support groups
Formal networks	Health providers, supporters, advocates	Community associations, patient groups	Members	May provide a range of information and support services to members. This may involve specialist and professional health providers. Example: Patient participation group, tenants' association
Community/voluntary organisations	Providers of services, supporters, advocates	Campaigning, delivering services, participating in working groups	Members, users, health professionals, health agencies	More formalised than networks and may have specific aims to provide services as well as support users. Example: MIND, SCOPE, RNID
Geographical communities	Polity, electors, providers, advocates	Voting, campaigning, developing networks between other groups	Health agencies, local authorities, government	Example: neighbourhood

Communities of interest (bracket label spanning Informal networks, Formal networks, and Community/voluntary organisations rows)

Individual and community health inequality

It is widely recognised that there are inequalities in health status, morbidity and mortality between deprived and affluent communities. However, the precise links between deprivation and health inequality are unclear and a range of characteristics is involved including individual, geographical and social factors. The relative effect of these will vary according to specific circumstances.

Early life factors and/or the cumulative effects of life events and effects of deprivation on social cohesion also play a significant role.[3,8] Thus, rather than blanket approaches applied the same way to everyone and all areas, developing approaches to reduce health inequalities will require:

- responding to individual circumstances
- addressing specific characteristics of local areas and communities.

Who produces and creates health?

There has tended to be little recognition of the role of the community in promoting its own health through community based action and community health initiatives.[9,10] It is clear that individuals, families and communities provide significant amounts of self-care and health prevention as illustrated in Table 4.1.[11,12]

Despite the continued importance of environmental health, housing, transport and education, public health has become dominated by the medical model and public health medicine promulgated by medical practitioners.[13,14] This has led to an emphasis on disease control and monitoring, epidemiological studies, individual health promotion and support to medical practitioners – most recently in relation to evidence-based medicine.

Nevertheless, it is widely recognised that most advances in health are the result of improvements in people's economic and social status – better housing, higher incomes, better education and so on. These improvements are not just the consequences of government intervention but derive from the actions of individuals, communities, organisations and international circumstances.

Moreover, as suggested above, social and community ties have been identified as important protective elements which promote health. Poor social relations appear to reduce resistance to a broad range of diseases and disabilities. This is not just an issue for individuals, as entire communities may be lacking in social connections.[3] Making sense of our lives, having control over our lives, and a dynamic approach to dealing with challenges have been identified as 'health-promoting'.

Recognition of the importance of healthy communities is reflected in current health policy with, for example, the creation of Health Action Zones (HAZs), Healthy Living Centres and Health Improvement Programmes. In particular, the new Primary Care Organisations (PCOs)* have been given the broad and ambitious brief to employ both individual and community approaches to address local health problems.

In adopting a more enlightened public health perspective, individuals and communities need to be seen as equal partners in promoting and producing health alongside many others. The medical and health professions are but one part of a range of individuals and organisations that have an impact on health, including local authorities, voluntary organisations and private companies and those that work within them.

Reconciling individual and community health

Primary care centre stage

If health is produced by both individuals and communities it makes sense to adopt methods of health needs assessment, health provision and health promotion at both individual and community levels. Of particular interest and potential are primary healthcare approaches to public health, given that primary care may have both a community and individual orientation.[13,16] There is good evidence to demonstrate that primary care can effectively contribute to individual health. For example, opportunistic GP advice to stop smoking reduces smoking rates, or GP advice on child safety coupled with provision of low cost safety equipment for families increases use of safety equipment and other safe practices.[15]

However, primary care in the UK has tended to focus on the individual at the expense of the community.[10] In redressing this balance a range of strategies and approaches have been developed, including community orientated primary care (COPC), rapid appraisal, community health needs assessment,

---

* Since 1997 in England the development of primary care has been focused on primary care groups – now primary care trusts (PCGs/PCTs) – who have gradually taken on the majority of healthcare services and public health functions. In Northern Ireland health boards currently retain most commissioning and public health functions, although there are proposals to develop English type PCTs. In Scotland non-commissioning PCTs have been developed with health boards retaining commissioning and strategic public health roles. In Wales there are local health groups that have a wider voluntary sector and local authority representation than in England, with the Welsh Assembly playing a stronger strategic public health role (see Peckham and Exworthy, 2003).[15]

Health for All, and community health projects.[17,18] More recently, government initiatives have promoted locality focused approaches to 'neighbourhood renewal'. In all these approaches the emphasis is on working with local communities.

Community orientated primary care

COPC has been described as '...the continual process by which primary healthcare teams* provide care to a defined community on the basis of its assessed health needs by the planned integration of public health with [primary care] practice'.[19] The idea originated in South Africa and Israel and has been supported by the World Health Organization and in the USA.[17] In 1992 the King's Fund established eight pilot practices in four sites in the UK – Northumberland, Sheffield, Winchester and Haringey.

COPC is an approach which involves primary care teams in identifying and prioritising, then assessing and addressing local health problems. Pilot practices in the UK addressed a range of problems including hypertension, urinary incontinence and the health of young people. More recent achievements have included a 'one stop' service for nursing, physiotherapy, chiropody and benefits advice for people over 75 years old and a benefits outreach service for older people in two London practices.[20]

COPC in the UK has tended to be a professionally led approach with little evidence that local community involvement or participation has been well developed within primary care.[10,21] The relationship between primary care and community development is discussed in Chapter 6. While COPC has not been taken up in any comprehensive way in the UK, the principles are embedded in current developments in local health needs assessment, which are considered below, and are being advocated as one approach to service development for new PCOs.[20]

Rapid appraisal

Rapid appraisal was developed by the World Health Organization for use in developing countries.[22] It involves identifying key local informants who have knowledge of their area. It has close links with the COPC approach and has been advocated by health professionals, including general practi-

---

* The primary healthcare team (PHCT) consists of the GPs, district and community nurses, health visitors and other staff working from general practice.

tioners, as one approach to identifying local health needs in defined 'natural' communities.[23] This is one step beyond the community diagnosis approach adopted in COPC but it still remains a professional-led exercise. Rather than being seen as a way of working with local communities, rapid appraisal has predominantly been used as a method for local health needs assessment with potential for planning local services. However it has led to locally based action undertaken as a partnership between residents and professionals (*see* Box 4.1).[23,24]

Box 4.1: Rapid appraisal in Dumbiedykes, Edinburgh

In the early 1990s members of the primary care team in Dumbiedykes undertook interviews of local residents. This identified a range of community issues with top priorities being the need for a bus service on the estate, creation of play areas and dog free zones and the opening of a supermarket nearby. In addition, suggestions were made to improve the running of general practices and the care of people with a mental illness. Following this research a health forum, comprising local residents and professionals who worked in the area, was established to seek action to meet these needs. The forum successfully achieved the top priorities and has strong inter-agency support. Further work was undertaken on mental health in the area and on incorporating community perspectives into the induction of new staff.

Community health needs assessment

Community health needs assessment is the identification of needs as expressed by local community members which may include health and non-health needs (*see* Box 4.1). This is also one of the key principles behind the production of local community care plans, which are joint plans prepared by social services in collaboration with health and voluntary agencies that identify local social care needs and how these are to be met. In health, needs assessment has been dominated by public health medicine.[10,14,25] Thus, while there are exceptions the majority of needs assessment is framed within a medical model. Lack of local accountability and community involvement has only served to reinforce such an approach. However there have been successful approaches which bring together epidemiological and community-based approaches such as in the West End Health Resource Centre in Newcastle (*see* Chapter 7). Promoting public participation and accountability at local level may contribute to social cohesion and improve needs assessment (*see* Chapters 6 and 7).

Community health movement

Community health action in the UK developed in the late 1970s with neighbourhood health projects set up by the Foundation for Alternatives. Other initiatives developed for specific communities of interest, such as refugees or women and children. They are characterised as self-determining, developing their own view of health needs and how they should be met.[26] By the mid-1980s there were thousands of local health groups[27] that were independent from healthcare services or working alongside them, demonstrating the ability of communities to engage in public health action.

The community health approach was widely supported by the 'Healthy City' and 'Health for All' movements.[28] The principles of participation, made explicit in the World Health Organization's *Health for All 2000*, emphasised the role of the community working with healthcare professionals, although the real level of participation in Healthy City/Health for All projects was often low.[9]

With its emphasis on self-defined needs and recognition of the broader environmental, material and social bases of inequalities in health,[7] the community health movement presented a challenge to Conservative government policy in the 1980s which did not adopt this broader perspective of health. For example, Edwina Curry, a Minister of Health, commented:

> 'I honestly don't think (health) has anything to do with poverty. The problem very often for many people is just ignorance … .and failing to realise they do have some control over their own lives'
> Quoted in Ranade, 1994, p.174.[29]

This individualistic approach to the public's health became reflected in a policy emphasis on the importance of personal lifestyle choices. Equity, community participation and inter-sectoral working were largely ignored in the Conservative government's response to the WHO's *Health for All*.[29]

Thus the development of community health projects in the 1980s and 1990s was marginalised and remained dependent on the goodwill and activity of individuals. Such initiatives largely developed alongside the NHS rather than as a mainstream part of healthcare services. Examples are outlined in Chapter 6.

Health Action Zones

Many of the principles of both Health for All and community health projects have been incorporated in the work of HAZs. These were developed from

1998 in 26 areas across England. They are based on developing strategic partnerships between health, local authorities and other partners in areas of deprivation and poor health to tackle health inequalities and modernise services through local innovation.

While HAZs themselves have covered large population areas they have predominantly fostered locally-based projects within communities which have addressed a range of issues including service provision, health needs assessment, community health development and education. Key principles which have underpinned the HAZ approach include achieving equity, engaging communities, developing partnership and adopting a person-centred approach to service delivery.

Community initiatives and primary care

Where community health initiatives worked alongside primary care, innovative responses to individual and community health have been developed. Examples of this include the Wells Park Health Project, which had a dramatic impact on the health of patients from the Wells Park Practice (*see* Box 4.2).[30]

Box 4.2: Wells Park Health Project

This project started in 1991 in the basement of the Wells Park Practice in Sydenham, Kent. The goals of the project were to promote health awareness and develop new approaches to primary care. While organisationally separate, the community health project and practice have formal and informal links through joint management committee and staff meetings.

The health project addressed health needs in different ways from the practice, using community-based solutions such as a reminiscence group for older people with depression, and campaigning for a bus to the local supermarket as a response to problems of angina. The practice has seen the project as an effective vehicle for health needs assessment. The project, by working with the practice, has also provided a basis for community participation and patient-centred care rooted in a wider social model of health rather than the medical model.[30]

More recently, the development of welfare advisory sessions has been supported by many practices as a way of dealing with individual patient problems but using a broader community perspective.[31] The use of advice workers in general practice has also been valuable for families with young children, with positive benefits for maternal and child health.[32] The roles of community health initiatives and community development in primary care are further considered in Chapter 6.

More recent policy initiatives

There has been a resurgence in community-based and -led initiatives[33] and a growing interest in community-based strategies.[34,35] New developments highlight community ownership and a holistic approach to health[36] which go beyond health services developments to incorporate strategies such as Building Better Communities (DETR), community co-ops, community cafés, LETS and 'time bank' schemes (*see* Box 4.3).[37]

Box 4.3: Rushey Green Time Bank

The time bank is closely related to the Local Exchange Trading Schemes where community members trade skills. In the time bank people trade hours of activity. There are a dozen or more time banks in the UK. One of these pioneering schemes was led by a GP in Rushey Green who saw the potential for time banks to have a health impact. He instigated a scheme in Rushey Green in 1999 which encourages local people to offer time to other local residents. Tasks on offer include story telling, fishing, odd jobs, babysitting and visiting elderly and housebound people.

Other recent policy initiatives drawing on community-based models include Sure Start and Healthy Living Centres or Networks. Sure Start is one of many community partnership approaches being developed in areas around the country. The approach was pioneered in the USA with each programme serving the local community 'within "pram pushing" distance'. The programme is targeted towards children and families in deprived circumstances, being delivered through local partnerships with the aim of providing a range of support services, including childcare, early learning and play opportunities, and support with parenting skills, as well as improved access to primary healthcare (*see* Box 4.4).

Box 4.4: Rose Hill – Littlemore Sure Start

The Sure Start project started in 1999 in an area of Oxford with the second largest 0–16-year-old population. The area also has the highest number of people reporting a limited long-term illness and high levels of unemployment. Rose Hill had a high proportion (25%) of children from Asian families on school roll and a high number of children on the special education needs register. There were no locally based health services in the area and few resources for under 4s and their families. The project has worked with local parents to establish a centre based at the First School for 0–3-year-olds, providing a community café, health clinics, crèche, playroom, etc. The project has also worked with the local Early Education Project. The focus of work is on prevention rather than crisis intervention. The project is a partnership between statutory and voluntary services and local families. There are parent representatives on the project group and research group which is conducting a local evaluation of the project.

Chapter 7 tells a further story about Sure Start from a local parent's perspective.

Neighbourhood renewal

Community-based approaches to health have been incorporated into a range of government policy programmes, including single regeneration budget (SRB), new deal for communities (NDC) and the neighbourhood renewal programme (NRA). The emphasis is on the need for local regeneration activity which engages local communities as citizens, service users and neighbours.[38]

The focus is on deprived neighbourhoods building on the experiences of previous programmes to improve local neighbourhoods so that '... within 10–20 years no one should be seriously disadvantaged by where they live' and to 'narrow the gap in [worklessness, crime, health, skills, housing and physical environment] measures between the most deprived neighbourhoods and the rest of the country'.[39] There is an attempt to join up policy initiatives across government – especially between local government and health. Increasingly, through local strategic partnerships, health agencies such as PCTs will be drawn into these programmes (*see* case examples in Chapter 6).

Challenges ahead

To date, PCOs have not found it easy to address public involvement.[40] When PCOs do attempt to involve the public it is from a more patient and service context rather than a broader public health perspective.[18] Taylor *et al.*[10] identified a number of barriers to effective public health activity including:

- lack of a 'shared language', i.e. shared definitions of public health, between primary care practitioners, and other stakeholders, including members of the community
- poor understanding of collaborative working both within primary health-care teams, and between GPs and other agencies
- the dominance of a medical model of primary care with its emphasis on general practice, and medically dominated organisation and values
- poor understanding of the key principles of public health among primary care professionals.

A cultural shift is needed (Meads *et al.*, 1999, p.47).[25] However, as Jennie Popay argued in her evidence to the House of Commons Health Committee, there are 'awesome' expectations now laid upon primary care to deliver the public health agenda and to address inequalities in health. She noted 'there is little if any evidence from research or practice that past primary care organisations or primary care medical professions have the capacity or the inclination to do this'.

Moreover, local people, especially those experiencing social deprivation, may not be able to prioritise public health issues, and may lack resources to participate actively in their communities. If they do get involved they may find it difficult to participate in conventional ways without support. There is a need for people in these communities to be empowered if they are to contribute as the government wishes.

PCOs will need to develop public health skills, and work together with other organisations, including local authorities, if they are to facilitate community contributions to public health. However, PCOs have a range of organisational and policy pressures that do not necessarily prioritise public health actions. Indeed, as PCTs in England absorb public health physicians from the dismantled health authorities, we may see an increased emphasis on medical approaches which may be at odds with the need to develop a *multi-disciplinary* public health workforce which works with local communities.

Conclusion

The implementation of government policy on public health will increasingly fall to primary care organisations and thus their role, and their relationships with local communities, will become more important in determining public health strategy and action. Involving the community in local public health issues within the context of developing local partnerships provides major challenges for PCOs. They are likely to find this area of work difficult and time consuming. Central to such an approach is the need for PCOs to develop a clearer understanding of public health and how to engage local people.[40]

Unfortunately, the time scales set by government for this work are unrealistic. Moreover, political imperatives will demand PCOs address other 'priorities' that will inevitably occupy their energies (for example, those of primary care service delivery or reducing hospital waiting lists and delays in patient discharges). This is likely to be at the expense of genuine and sustainable primary and community development. Real change will rely on time, commitment and persistence.

References

1 DoH (1999) *Saving Lives: Our Healthier Nation.* Cm4386. The Stationery Office, London.

2 DoH (2002) *Shifting the Balance of Power: Next Steps.* The Stationery Office, London.

3 Wilkinson RG (1996) *Unhealthy Societies: the affliction of inequality.* Routledge, London.

4 Gaskin K and Vincent J (1996) *Co-operating for Health.* CRSP, Loughborough University, Loughborough.

5 Putnam RD (1995) Tuning In, Turning Out: the strange disappearance of social capital in America. *Political Science and Politics*, pp. 664–83. December.

6 DoH (1997) *The New NHS: Modern, Dependable.* Cm3807. The Stationery Office, London.

7 Townsend P, Davidson N and Whitehead M (1992) *Inequalities in Health.* Penguin, Harmandsworth.

8 Wilkinson RG (1997) Health inequalities: relative or absolute material standards? *BMJ.* **314**: 591–5.

9 Petersen A and Lupton D (1996) *The New Public Health.* Sage, London.

10 Taylor P, Peckham S and Turton P (1998) *A Public Health Model of Primary Care: from concept to reality.* Public Health Alliance, Birmingham.

11 WHO/UNICEF (1978) *Primary Health Care: The Alma Ata Conference.* WHO, Geneva.

12 Zakus JDL and Lysack CL (1998) Revisiting community participation. *Health Policy Plan.* **13**(1): 1–12.

13 Macdonald J (1993) *Primary Health Care: medicine in its place.* Earthscan, London.

14 Baggott R (2000) *The Politics of Public Health.* MacMillan, Basingstoke.

15 Peckham S and Exworthy M (2003) *Primary Care in the UK: policy, organisation and management.* Palgrave/Macmillian, Basingstoke.

16 Starfield B (1998) *Primary Care: balancing health needs services and technology.* Oxford University Press, Oxford.

17 Gillam S and Miller R (1997) *COPC – A Public Health Experiment in Primary Care.* King's Fund, London.

18 Lupton C, Peckham S and Taylor P (1998) *Managing Public Involvement in Healthcare Purchasing.* Open University Press, Buckingham.

19 Gillam S, Plamping D, McClenahan J, *et al.* (1994) *Community Oriented Primary Care.* King's Fund, London.

20 Iliffe S and Leniham P (2003) Integrated primary care and public health: learning from the community-oriented primary care model. *Int J Health Serv.* **33**(1): 85–98.

21 Peckham S, Macdonald J and Taylor P (1996) *Towards a Public Health Model of Primary Care.* First report of the public health and primary care project. Public Health Alliance, Birmingham.

22 World Health Organization (1992) *Guidelines for Rapid Appraisal to Assess Community Health Needs.* WHO, Geneva.

23 Murray SA (1999) Experiences with 'rapid appraisal' in primary care: involving the public in assessing health needs, orientating staff, and educating medical students. *BMJ.* **318**: 440–4.

24 Ong BN, Humphris G, Annett H and Rifkin S (1991) Rapid appraisal in an urban setting – an example from the developed world. *Soc Sci Med.* **32**(8): 909–15.

25 Meads G, Killoran A, Ashcroft J and Cornish Y (1999) *Mixing Oil and Water: How can primary care organisations improve health as well as deliver effective health care?* HEA, London.

26 Dun R (1991) Working with the voluntary sector. In: A McNaught (ed) *Managing Community Health Services.* Chapman Hall, London.

27 Kenner C (1986) *Community Health Action.* Bedford Square Press, London.

28 Ashton J and Seymour H (1988) *The new Public Health.* Open University Press, Milton Keynes.

29 Ranade W (1994) *A Future for the NHS? Health Care for the Millennium.* Longman, Harlow.

30 Fisher B (1994) The Wells Park Health Project. In: Z Heritage (ed.) *Community Participation in Primary Care.* Occasional Paper 64. RCGP, London.

31 Abbott S and Hobby L (2000) Welfare benefits advice in primary care: evidence of improvements in health. *Public Health.* **114**(5): 324–27.

32   Reading R, Steel S and Reynolds S (2002) Citizens advice in primary care for families with young children. *Child Care Health Development.* **28**(1): 39–45.

33   Smithies J and Webster G (1998) *Community Involvement in Health. From Passive Recipients to Active Participants.* Arena, Aldershot.

34   Demos (1997) *Escaping Poverty. From Safety Nets to Networks of Opportunity.* Demos, London.

35   New Economics Foundation (undated) *Participation Works! 21 Techniques of Community Participation for the 21st Century.* NEF with UK Community Participation Network, London.

36   Gaskin K, Vincent J and Miles A (1998) *Healthy Living Centres. Practical Illustrations of Key Principals.* CRSP, Loughborough University, Loughborough.

37   Cowe R (2000) Swap Shop. *The Guardian.* 30 August.

38   Audit Commission (2002) *Policy Focus: Neighbourhood Renewal.* Audit Commission, London.

39   Social Exclusion Unit (2001) A New Commitment to Neighbourhood Renewal – National Strategy Action Plan. SEU, London.

40   Anderson W, Florin D, Mountford L and Gillam S (2002) *Every Voice Counts: primary care organisations and public involvement.* King's Fund, London.

CHAPTER 5

Sustaining a healthy workforce

Jenny Firth-Cozens

Introduction

Health service staff have considerably higher levels of stress than other workers in Britain,[1] while doctors in particular have higher stress, depression and alcoholism than other professional groups. A study of general practitioners showed 17% above the threshold for depression[2] and 33% above the threshold for stress.[3] Similarly, nurses have been found to have a high risk of physical illness, mental ill health and suicide,[4] though most studies take place in secondary care settings. Other primary care staff have not been studied, though health service managers as a whole have been found to have 33% above the threshold for stress, compared to 22% of British managers in general.[1] The changes that primary care is currently experiencing are likely to exacerbate these symptoms across all staff, as is working in a disadvantaged area.

This is not only an important issue for the individual staff and the teams to which they belong. It is also a crucial factor in providing good quality care to patients, since considerable research has described the ways that the stress, fatigue and dissatisfaction of doctors impact negatively upon patient care.[5] In addition, recruitment and retention of staff lower the quality of care, and stress is one of the main precipitants of the dissatisfaction that leads to early retirement.[6] This chapter will focus upon interventions for stress – the ways that staff can care for themselves and for their colleagues.

Causes of stress

Many of the job-related causes of stress in primary care are no different to those seen in other organisations, e.g. role overload, difficulties with superiors, role conflict (i.e., between family and work), and low participation and control in non-medical staff.[7] Role ambiguity is another common cause of stress in the workplace, involving not knowing when you have done enough or done a good job, and also being unclear about the boundaries of your role and those of others. In this sense medicine in particular has many uncertainties attached to it, often without the chance to discuss these through supervision or even peer review.

There is sometimes little appreciation of the roles of others within the team, and this has been shown to be the case especially with doctors.[8] Poor relationships with the boss has been indicated through meta-analysis as the greatest cause of stress across numerous situations in various types of organisation.[9] In medicine as a whole, longitudinal research[10] shows that abusive relationships in the workplace, interacting with a vulnerable personality, are, over time, the best predictors of alcohol abuse. It is clear from a number of studies that doctors in particular greatly underestimate the effects, for better or for worse, that they can have on their colleagues.

Within general practice most research has been conducted with medical staff and findings suggest that the patients themselves are one of the greatest sources of stress, along with difficulties with partners, fear of litigation and fear of violence.[11] Howie and Porter's work in Edinburgh[12] shows that a quick consulting rate not only creates lower patient satisfaction, and so is more likely to increase frustration and difficult relationships between staff and patients, but also creates more stress to those GPs who are more 'patient-centred'.

Working in deprived communities

Patients within disadvantaged areas are likely to have higher levels of stress and depression themselves and to experience far more difficulties within their lives than are possible to address within the clinical setting, and this will reduce staff's sense of control and usefulness. There is inevitably a higher rate of violence, and the fear of this, particularly when on call, becomes a much more salient stressor within these areas of deprivation. Being on call at night is a clear stressor, perhaps partly linked to the threat of violence, but also because in numerous studies a lack of sleep is related to higher depressive symptoms.[13]

Individuals also bring to the workplace aspects of personality or life events which make them more vulnerable to stress, depression or physical health risks in general or at certain times. For example, the Type A personality (characterised by competitive, driving, intense, controlling, impatient and hostile behaviours) is often rewarded in our workplaces but is a risk factor for coronary heart disease, particularly the behaviours relating to hostility.[14] Characteristics can interact with the workplace to create psychological problems. For example, as described above, GPs who take longer with patients have higher stress levels if they are having to work more briefly than they would prefer.[11]

For doctors who have chosen to work in disadvantaged areas where presenting problems are often so much more complex than in other places, having to work at an unsuitably fast pace is likely to become a particular conflict with their value systems. Moreover, opportunities to help their patients in any major way against the outside forces of poor housing, transport, education, drug use and high violence are minimal, and this may add to their frustrations.

Factors influencing stress and depression

In my own longitudinal study of general practitioners, the two main predictors of depression over ten years were high self-criticism as students and reports of early sibling rivalry.[2] It is clear that being a very self-critical doctor might be good for the patients but the uncertainty and error that are inevitable within medicine make life hard if you consistently take responsibility for all that goes wrong. Moreover, such doctors might blame themselves for their apparent inability to bring about major change in their patients' difficult lives.

All this is likely to be exacerbated as the status of professionals in general and doctors in particular becomes lower, and as patients challenge more and are clearly less grateful for what they receive. On the other hand, those who are very low in self-criticism and are more likely to blame others than themselves, have more difficult relationships with their patients.[11] Like so many things in life, the aim for health is to be somewhere in between, taking legitimate responsibility where appropriate.

Finally, although it may seem difficult to change, early family relationships do play a role in the workplace.[15] Current depression in general practitioners[2] was also predicted by poor sibling relationships which, taken alongside the considerable partnership problems experienced in general practice (and often seen as due to inequalities amongst the partners), suggests that having unresolved early family conflicts may interact with the workplace 'family' in adulthood.

Within nursing and medicine and also more generally, individual coping styles involving denial and avoidance of stressors have been found predictive of stress.[16,17] In addition, there will be times when life events, especially those involving loss, happen to all staff and this is always a time of extra vulnerability. For example, it is much more difficult for staff to deal with distressed or dying patients when they have recently suffered similarly with someone close.

Likewise, a lack of social support at home can be particularly difficult if there is also inadequate support at work. This can make those who are working in the community particularly vulnerable, since it is always more difficult for them to feel part of the team. Within healthcare, those who are in good teams have significantly lower stress than those in poor teams or no teams at all,[18] and there is also evidence that those who regard the team they belong to as multi-disciplinary also have lower stress levels,[19] probably because they can share skills and look for support from a wider group than just their own profession. However, most primary care teams do not meet the criteria of 'good teamworking'.[20]

These stressors are summarised in Table 5.1.

Table 5.1: Job-related and individual stressors in the workplace, particularly in general practice

Job-related stressors	Individual stressors
Overload and sleep loss.	Coping through denial or avoidance.
Role conflict.	Life events, particularly involving loss.
High responsibility for people.	Lack of social support.
Role ambiguity.	Type A behaviour pattern.
Difficult relationships, especially with superiors.	
Low participation and discretion.	*In addition, within primary care:*
Low occupational support.	High self-criticism.
	Patient-centred approach.
In addition, within primary care:	Conflict of career with personal life.
	Early family relationships.
Difficult patients.	
Distressed relatives.	
Making mistakes.	
On call.	
Fear of litigation, and actual complaints and claims.	
Fear of violence.	

Interventions in primary care

Interventions to deal with stress within organisations and teams can be primary or preventive, or they can be secondary – directed at alleviating stress and other psychological problems when they occur. Like all good public health, the more that can actually be prevented, the better, but many organisations tend to opt for secondary care only, for example by providing sick leave, early retirement, and access to counselling but not addressing the causes of the problem organisationally.

There are few methodologically rigorous studies of organisational interventions. However, one study does meet the criteria.[21] There, the authors used a sample of 22 hospitals for the intervention and compared these with 22 control hospitals matched in terms of being urban or rural and the number of previous claims. The intervention involved entirely preventive strategies using a variety of organisational interventions alongside brief stress management training for staff. Over the year of the trial, litigation claims in the 22 intervention hospitals reduced by 70%, compared to the control hospitals where claims stayed the same. In this part of the chapter I shall address both preventive and secondary interventions for stress, targeting the organisation and the individual.

Organisational strategies

Underlying most useful interventions, an organisational culture needs to be developed which accepts that stress is a serious and sometimes inevitable part of working life, particularly within healthcare and in areas of high deprivation. Regarding stressed workers as anomalies rather than people with a very normal reaction to difficult and demanding work will not be useful.

The second important task for an organisation is to ensure excellent two-way communication so that all layers of staff can have their voices heard. This is important both as a means to increase participation in decision making, which in turn raises well being,[22] and also to improve patient care, because staff are the experts in seeing when things are going wrong. An open door for such messages raises morale in general as well as taking warnings out of the whistle-blowing context and into the culture that there is a duty to improve care.

Accurate communication to staff makes them aware of the organisation's pathway, successes and difficulties and this again allows a sense of belonging, increases participation in addressing problems, builds trust and reduces rumours which are a symptom of poor organisational health. Full participation in decision making within teams is a key factor in Murphy's review of organisational interventions for health service stress.[23]

The organisation also has an important educational role, partly through creating a culture which encourages learning from experience, but also in providing appropriate training for staff. Training in stress management has been shown to be effective both for staff and indirectly for their patients,[24] but development programmes will also be necessary in the areas of team leadership, assertiveness training, problem-solving techniques, dealing with difficult people – patients and their relatives as well as colleagues – and handling violence.

Organisations within primary care are growing too large to address more than these underlying cultural, structural and training issues. Beyond such overarching considerations it is the team level which will provide the most appropriate means of creating a healthy workforce, and the organisation needs to put real effort into developing good team leaders and finding the means to reward and support its team structure.

At primary care team level

Good teamworking is increasingly being shown as an excellent way of lowering stress levels and also of improving the quality of care.[25] Teams that meet regularly are clear about their team goal and individual members' roles, and those that have good communication within and outwith the team can provide the support needed to deal with difficult patients and complaints, to balance family and work, to handle uncertainty and ambiguity, and to increase participation. In addition, as a mini-organisation in itself such a team can address operational problems surrounding consulting times, on-call rotas, etc., so that types of patient are more appropriately balanced for different types of clinical skills, and staff who are in any way facing difficult times in their lives can be protected as necessary.

Good team leaders may occasionally be born that way, but most need training in both leadership and management skills. In Australia the provision of a small booklet on how to manage people in ways that reduce their stress (that is, to manage them well) has contributed significantly to the dramatic reduction in claims for workers' compensation for job-related psychological distress.[26] Clearly such preventive measures are well worth doing. Good team leaders can also affect the quality of work the team produces; in other words they can improve patient care.[25]

Finally, organisations can provide secondary interventions through access to counselling and psychotherapy services, whether in-house or externally provided. These need to be linked to management in ways which allow presenting problems accumulating from individual staff and demonstrating a pattern of poor organisational practice to be recognised and addressed. If this is not done, organisations can ignore these difficulties by using a counselling service as a sponge to soak up staff distress, and do nothing to rectify fundamental problems.

Individual interventions

Preventive measures for individuals come under the broad umbrella of stress management skills. First and foremost, they include some form of relaxation technique and, if possible, some form of exercise, both of which, with regular practice can bring long lasting benefits to both psychological and physical health.[27,28] The other central area of intervention is around cognitive restructuring. This encourages people to challenge the causes they make for things (for example, that they are responsible for everything that goes wrong, but nothing that goes right; or that this event is going to affect everything in their lives for ever) and accept that they cannot control everything, but that there are areas where they can bring about change.

Coping skills training includes these strategies but also encourages the use of social support, assertiveness, time management and problem solving. On the other hand, it warns against using dangerous strategies such as alcohol abuse for chronic stress, or denial and avoidance as a way to cope with distressing events. These events are an inevitable part of healthcare, as well as being a feature of most people's personal lives at some point.

It is important that healthcare workers are not seen as being so strong and resourceful that they can deal intuitively with such distress.[29] In fact, there is evidence that writing or talking about such an event significantly reduces attendance at health centres over the following year, so it seems that physical as well as psychological health is also improved when emotional reactions to events are discussed.[30,31] Another poor coping strategy is bad behaviour; although it needs challenging, it is also important to realise that it is often a way of showing misery, especially in men.[32] A good team leader will recognise the need for providing a forum where these issues can be addressed.

People will need extra support if they are going through difficult life events such as separation or serious family illnesses. These occasions take their toll on the individuals concerned but also inevitably on their patient care. In terms of chronic stress, working mothers who are hospital doctors have significantly higher symptom levels than childless women doctors, while having children appears to make no difference at all to the stress levels of men.[32] As the proportion of women entering medicine begins to exceed that of men, this issue can no longer be ignored, and making working life more tolerable for mothers as well as fathers must be a priority.

Stress management techniques and extra team support at certain times of our lives are likely to help most people stay healthy within the workplace. However, at times a proportion of staff will need more professional help to stop problems developing more seriously or to alleviate them when they become clinical conditions. Whether this is counselling for more focused problems such as divorce or family problems, or whether the services of clinical psychology, psychotherapy or psychiatry are necessary will depend upon the severity of the problem.

There is evidence that brief psychological interventions for job-related stress and clinical depression not only reduce symptom levels significantly but also create more positive perceptions of the workplace.[33] The addresses of places to go for this help (and also for voluntary agencies such as Alcoholics Anonymous and Relate) should be a prominent part of the practice noticeboard so that people not only know where to go without needing to ask, but also so that they can see that the organisation accepts such problems are a part of everyone's life, and can be remedied.

A programme like this – both organisational and individual – is not a one-off initiative but is ongoing, an essential part of management in terms of normal health and safety. It benefits not only the staff concerned but also raises the quality of care for the patients they treat, and so the leaders of health organisations should be judged, at least in part, on the well being of those they employ.

References

1   Wall TD, Bolden RI, Borril CS, et al. (1997) Minor psychiatric disorders in NHS trust staff: occupational and gender differences. B J Psychiatry. **171**: 519–23.

2   Firth-Cozens J (1998) Individual and organisational predictors of depression in general practitioners. Br J Gen Pract. **48**: 1647–51.

3   Firth-Cozens J (1997) Predicting stress in general practitioners: 10 year follow up postal survey. BMJ. **315**: 34–5.

4   Baldwin P (1999) Stress in nurses. In: J Firth-Cozens and RL Payne (eds) Stress in Health Professionals. John Wiley, Chichester.

5   Firth-Cozens J (2001) Interventions to improve physicians' wellbeing and patient care. Soc Sci Med. **52**: 215–22.

6   Luce A, van Zwanenberg T, Firth-Cozens J and Tinwell C (2002) What might encourage later retirement among general practitioners? J Manag Med. **16**: 303–10.

7   Schuler RS (1984) Organizational stress and coping: a model and overview. In: AS Sethi and RS Schuler (eds) Handbook of Organizational Stress Coping Strategies. Ballinger, Cambridge, Massachusetts.

8   Bond J, Cartilidge AM, Gregson BA, et al. (1985) A study of interprofessional collaboration in primary health care organisations. University of Newcastle upon Tyne, Health Care Research, Newcastle upon Tyne.

9   Hogan R, Curphy GJ, Hogan J (1994) What we know about leadership. Am Psych. **49**(6): 493–504.

10   Richman JA, Flaherty JA and Rospenda KM (1996) Perceived workplace harassment experiences and problem drinking among physicians: broadening the stress/alienation paradigm. *Addiction.* **91**(3): 391–403.

11   Firth-Cozens J (1995) Sources of stress in junior doctors and general practitioners. *Yorkshire Medicine.* **7**: 10–13.

12   Howie JGR and Porter M (1999) Stress in general practitioners. In: J Firth-Cozens and RL Payne (eds) *Stress in Health Professionals.* John Wiley, Chichester.

13   Firth-Cozens J and Cording H (1993) Do doctors' hours of work and sleep affect the quality of patient care? *Qual Saf Health Care* (in press).

14   Smith T and Pope M (1990) Cynical hostility as a health risk: current status and future directions. *Social Behavior and Personality.* **5**: 77–8.

15   Malan DH (1979) *Individual Psychotherapy and the Science of Psycho-dynamics.* Butterworths, London.

16   Tyler P and Cushway D (1992) Stress, coping and mental wellbeing in hospital nurses. *Stress Medicine.* **8**: 91–8.

17   Koeske GF, Kirk SA and Koeske RD (1993) Coping with job stress: which strategies work best? *J Occup Organ Psychol.* **66**: 319–35.

18   Carter AJ and West MA (1999) Sharing the burden – team work in health care settings. In: J Firth-Cozens and RL Payne (eds) *Stress in Health Professionals.* John Wiley, Chichester.

19   Firth-Cozens J, Moss F, Rayner K and Paice E (2000) The effect of 1-year rotations on stress in pre-registration house officers. *Hospital medicine.* **61**: 859–60.

20   West MA and Poulton BC (1997) A failure of function: teamwork in primary health care. *J Interprof Care.* **11**(2): 205–16.

21   Jones JW, Barge BN, Steffy BD, *et al.* (1988) Stress and medical malpractice: organizational risk assessment and intervention. *J Appl Psychol.* **4**: 727–35.

22   Wall I and Clegg C (1981) A longitudinal study of group work redesign. *J Occup Behavior.* **2**: 31–49.

23   Murphy L (1999) Organisational interventions to reduce stress in health care professionals. In: J Firth-Cozens and RL Payne (eds) *Stress in Health Professionals.* John Wiley, Chichester.

24   Firth-Cozens J (2001) Teams, culture and managing risk. In: C Vincent (ed) *Clinical Risk Management* (2e). BMJ Books, London.

25   Stanton M (1999) Occupational Stress: Australian Approaches. Paper given at the *Work Stress and Health '99: Organization of Work in a Global Economy conference.* American Psychological Association, Baltimore.

26   Ross R and Altmaier E (1994) *Intervention in Occupational Stress.* Sage, London.

27   Roskies E (1987) *Stress Management for the Health Type A.* Guilford Press, New York.

28   Luce A, Firth-Cozens J, Midgley S and Burges C (2002) After the Omagh Bomb: Posttraumatic Stress Disorder in Health Service Staff. *J Trauma Stress.* **17**(1): 27–30.

29   Esterling BA, Antoni M, Kumar M, *et al.* (1990) Emotional repression, stress disclosure responses, and Epstein-Barr viral capsid antigen titers. *Psychosom Med.* **52**: 397–410.

30   Pennebaker JW, Kiecolt-Glaser J, Glaser R (1988) Disclosure of traumas and immune function: health implications for psychotherapy. *J Consult Clin Psychol.* **56**: 239–45.

31   Block J and Gjerde P (1991) Personality antecedents of depressive tendencies in 18 year olds. *J Pers Soc Psychol.* **60**(5): 726–38.

32   Firth-Cozens J, Bonanno D and Redfern N (2000) *What is Training Like?* University of Northumbria at Newcastle, Newcastle upon Tyne.

33   Firth-Cozens J and Hardy G (1992) Occupational stress, clinical treatment and changes in job perceptions. *J Occup Organ Psychol.* **65**: 81–8.

CHAPTER 6

Community development and primary healthcare

Jan Smithies

Introduction

Chapter 4 provided an overview of community oriented approaches to health. This chapter considers the principles of community development (CD) and its relation with primary care more closely, offering examples of this in practice. CD has often focused its activity at primary healthcare levels. However it has not necessarily worked with or through primary healthcare professionals.

One of the earliest examples of CD work in primary care is the Pioneer Health Centre in Peckham.[1] This work came about through the recognition by two GPs that their patients' ill health was largely a result of the social conditions they were living in. The centre they opened in 1935 included a whole range of recreational, nutritional, educational and social activities as well as health services.

Nearly 70 years on their early vision is being translated into the concept of 'healthy living centres' (HLCs).[2] This approach might be described as linking public health and primary care. However, as highlighted in Chapter 4, the medical model which has underpinned definitions of primary care and public health has inhibited the development of a community perspective on health.

Opportunities ahead

Through the establishment of Primary Care Trusts (PCTs), primary care has become a central focus for health resources and decision making in terms of government policy and its practical implementation. They are increasingly identifying local health needs and priorities, and planning and securing services to meet those needs. PCTs are particularly important within local communities because of the range of partnership initiatives which are seeking to engage them in local projects to tackle regeneration, social exclusion and health inequalities.

Primary healthcare workers, both as individual practitioners and collectively through PCTs, are being asked and expected to play a part in bringing about large-scale social change. The stiff challenge for PCTs is to improve health and address inequalities within their communities, not simply to commission health services.[3]

As we shall see later in this chapter, CD is fundamentally about ways of bringing about change through the empowerment of local people and communities. While it has been suggested that 'the principles of change management are poorly understood in primary care',[4] CD can be a way of supporting primary care practitioners, teams and PCTs in breaking through the barriers to change.

What is community development?

A recent definition emphasises the issue of power:

> 'CD is about building active and sustainable communities based on social justice and mutual respect. It is about changing power structures to remove the barriers that prevent people from participating in the issues that affect their lives. Community workers support individuals, groups and organisations in this process...'[5]

Yet, translating a definition of CD into real lives, in varied communities, engaging with a myriad of professionals, organisations and wider societal and policy influences, is more complex than this short definition would suggest. CD has recently been strengthened by the government's broader policy frameworks which recognise its role and understand its contribution.

What is a community?

Notions of community are considered in Chapter 4. Most of us are likely to be part of a number of different communities at any given time, the concept is not static and the community we belong to will change over time. For example, a community may be something that people choose for themselves so that they feel a part of something (a cultural group for example) or it may be simply an administrative concept such as a PCT catchment area.

Community development values

Although the methods adopted by community organisations and CD workers may vary widely, there are shared values and principles outlined in Boxes 6.1 and 6.2.

Box 6.1: Values of community development[5]

- Social justice – enabling people to claim their human rights, meet their needs and have greater control over the decision-making processes which affect their lives.
- Participation – facilitating democratic involvement by people in the issues which affect their lives based on full citizenship, autonomy, and shared power, skills, knowledge and experience.
- Equality – challenging the attitudes of individuals, and the practices of institutions and society, which discriminate against and marginalise people.
- Learning – recognising the skills, knowledge and expertise that people contribute and develop by taking action to tackle social, economic, political and environmental problems.
- Co-operation – working together to identify and implement action, based on mutual respect of diverse cultures and contributions.

CD has three main features that separate it out from other forms of community-based work.[6] Part of the challenge of CD is combining all three aspects in work with local communities, but also with local agencies and professionals.

Box 6.2: Main features of community development

- Challenging social exclusion, poverty, disadvantage and discrimination.
- Strengthening communities by work that enables full citizenship, community-led collective action, participative democracy, empowerment, problem-focused learning and preventative action.
- Influencing policy through community involvement, collaboration and community-led agendas.

Who gets involved in community development?

Communities themselves are the main stakeholders in any CD activity, bringing skills, expertise, contacts and personal commitment and energy. National government are stakeholders, through their policy and funding priorities. Local public sector organisations often provide the local policy environment and sometimes the resource infrastructure. National bodies like the lottery or local charitable trusts or private sector funders may also be stakeholders. Both statutory and voluntary sector organisations are often involved in direct work with local communities in relation to the training, organisational and administrative support they need to organise effective community groups and campaigns.

Community development and health

CD and health projects have a long history.[7] However, certain common principles and goals have endured, and still underpin CD and health initiatives, including:

- a positive view of health
- a collective approach to the social causes of ill health
- better access for people to health information and resources
- increased self confidence amongst people
- better relationships between clients and health professionals
- greater public influence over health policies and allocation of resources.

Social exclusion: involving communities

Social exclusion is the result of '...complex connections between causes and symptoms of deprivation and exclusion...'[8] Good health is an integral part of social inclusion. Poor health is both a factor that can contribute to social exclusion and one of the likely consequences of social exclusion. Strong communities are seen as 'vital to an inclusive society'. However, it is important that communities are listened to:

> 'One of the reasons that single issue approaches fail is that they are conceived by those responsible for a single function as a solution to problems which are multi-dimensional. Often the only people who understand all those dimensions are those who experience them – the excluded community. For this reason it is essential that communities

are placed at the heart of decision making about initiatives being designed for their benefit.'[8]

Community development or community based?

There is confusion between CD approaches and community based approaches to health promotion. The latter can be seen as 'top-down', and often 'the size of the effects has been meagre in relation to the effort expended.'[9] For example, a 1990s review of 135 disease prevention community based programmes in the USA found that they failed to reach the most disadvantaged people, or to engage their participation in programme planning, implementation and evaluation. They tended to focus on only one set of behavioural risk factors or concerns, such as HIV, cardiovascular disease, substance abuse or violence, rather than the social and economic factors that render these inter-related problems for the health of urban populations. They also often failed to draw upon any theoretical behavioural or social science models for the changes they sought.[10]

In contrast, CD may impact on health at three broad levels:[11]

1 The personal impact on people involved through:
   - encouraging people to adopt a critical and reflective stance in relation to the issues that affect them, e.g. the development of a lesbian, gay and bi-sexual 'communities of interest' dimension to Bradford's Neighbourhood Renewal Strategy – brought together by these communities themselves with CD support
   - explicit aims to include people who are otherwise marginalised or ignored by mainstream services, e.g. CD support to South Asian communities and groups to ensure their lead role in a successful New Opportunities Fund (NOF) Healthy Living Centre bid in Huddersfield
   - individual involvement in collective action which can build social networks and a sense of purpose and achievement, e.g. a community campaign for play spaces and equipment for local children in Haworth, West Yorkshire.

2 Outcomes from specific CD activities:
   - tackling health issues originating through community concerns such as mental health, drugs, food and diet, women's health, environmental issues, quality of local health services
   - tackling other issues with a public health impact such as anti-poverty work, community economic development, youth and environmental work

- reorienting policies and priorities of agencies defined through consultation and involvement of local communities leading to the development of services that are better targeted to local need.

3 General outcomes through community development's contribution to stronger communities that are sustainable, equitable and liveable, e.g. major regeneration initiatives encompassing employment, housing, health, social and economic dimensions, such as the Wythenshaw Partnership in Manchester who build CD into all aspects of their work, with a particular focus on young people.

Depending on how widely we understand the concept of primary care, all of the above can be seen to contribute towards preventing ill health, promoting well being and allowing all individuals to fulfil their health potential.

Community development and primary care

The following considers CD and primary care in relation to needs assessment, consultation and involving the public, the role of primary care professionals and how CD can facilitate delivery of primary care.

PCTs and public involvement

Public involvement is a key role and responsibility for PCTs underscored by the Department of Health for their PCG predecessors:

> 'The whole ethos of PCGs should be open and involving ... [DOH Guidance] is clear that the views of all those that have an interest should be represented ... PCGs are required to demonstrate how they will involve people and disseminate information.
>
>   User and public involvement should be regarded as an integral part of a PCG's activities. It should not be seen as an add on, nor as being fulfilled by a one off activity such as an annual meeting. The aim should be continuous dialogue with communities.'[12]

There is a danger of this role being seen solely as the function of PCT lay members who can become marginalised if their role is ill defined or unsupported. However, engaging with the community should be the business of every board member. There are several publications suggesting how to involve the public in the NHS e.g. NHS Executive (2000).[13] However, using methods such as focus groups, community surveys or open meetings will often only reach highly motivated people already engaged in community activity.

CD is also about enabling the involvement of the most socially excluded members of society. It is not a 'quick fix' solution, but an approach which takes time in order to build up relationships, trust, 'community capacity', i.e. the individual and collective skills, knowledge and confidence that are needed for people to play a full and active part in their own communities, and 'community infrastructure', i.e. the formal and informal networks, groups and resources that enable people to come together to take collective decisions and action.

Case example: Wakefield

Against a background of CD work supported by the Wakefield Health Action Zone, the local voluntary sector and regeneration partnerships, Eastern Wakefield PCT is working to build up primary care practice and service specific community involvement strategies (e.g. community nursing, school nursing) led through the trust's Patient Liaison and Information Service (PALS) and a trust CD framework, led by the trust's dedicated senior public health manager (*see* Box 6.3).

The PCT has 'inherited' a successful £1 million 'Healthy Living Centre' in

---

Box 6.3: PCT approach to CD in Eastern Wakefield

- Draw up strategies for action that are endorsed and owned by the PCT board and staff.
- Achieve clarity about roles and resource needs.
- Map all the different community initiatives that exist district wide and within the PCT's catchment area.
- Develop user-friendly information about the role of PCTs.
- Develop training and professional development initiatives to widen knowledge of CD and CD skills within the wide range of primary care professionals linked to the PCT.
- Work with CD workers and initiatives in outreach to community groups, organisations and gathering places to get their involvement in shaping the trust's work.
- Offer skilled, dedicated CD support to communities to enable them to develop their own groups' resources and local action on issues of concern.
- Undertake this work in partnership with other key bodies and sectors.

---

one of its localities from work undertaken, prior to the PCT coming into existence, by local people and the HAZ CD workers. It also has a team of nine CD workers, plus a team manager, brought together from localities within the PCT area, who are funded from short-term sources, such as SRB, Neighbourhood Renewal Fund and the HAZ.

Role of PCTs and primary care professionals in CD initiatives

Funding and commissioning

CD and public involvement cost money. Even properly organised one-off consultation events need adequate financing, particularly ones that aim at involving people who need additional support to participate. They might include, for example, transport for older people, sign language interpreters, readers for blind people, sitters for carers, translation of materials for non-English speakers.

CD and health projects have often been funded through special area based schemes such as the SRB or one of the lottery funds. However, most of these schemes require evidence of 'matched funding'. Increasingly this will fall to PCTs in replacing past health or local authority support to community health initiatives. Some PCTs are allocating mainstream resources to establish their own internal CD teams; others are commissioning voluntary or community organisations, or local partnerships, to take forward CD work.

Fostering CD skills amongst primary care team members

A whole range of practitioners ranging from GPs to pharmacists to dietitians have been involved in CD health projects. In some cases whole practices work in partnership with CD and health projects within the same premises (*see* Wells Park Practice, discussed in Chapter 4). Health visitors perhaps have the greatest profile, their professional organisation has its own national CD Group.[14]

Pauline Craig, a health visitor in Drumchapel, Glasgow saw her role as enabling and supporting people to articulate their own and their community's needs; assisting people to develop personal abilities and coping mechanisms;

setting up support networks; improving access to health information and working for change in health related policies and strategies.[15]

'Health professionals may need to relinquish established attitudes and behaviours in order to encourage the contributions of local people.'[4]

Better training may help. For example, exposing medical students to the complexities of inner city and housing estate life through local community work placements.[16] The benefits of such schemes have included students contributing to local research and information for health promotion, gaining experience of community participation and inter-agency partnership working, and enhanced understanding of social/economic/political determinants of health.

Involvement in partnership work

There is no shortage of opportunities for PCTs and primary care professionals to get involved in strategic and practical initiatives for health improvement, for example in Local Strategic Partnerships, which are the umbrella bodies bringing together all key local stakeholders across a given area (usually a local authority boundary).

Relevant partnership initiatives, which can contribute towards PCTs' ability to meet their responsibilities to reduce health inequalities, include Health Improvement Programmes, Health Action Zones, Healthy Living Centres, Community Safety Strategies, Community Plans (being drawn up by all local authorities), Single Regeneration Budget and New Deal for Communities regeneration initiatives, Neighbourhood Renewal and Sure Start.

All of these offer opportunities to:

- access additional funding and other resources, and the opportunity to more effectively pool and channel existing resources
- bring together a wider range of skills and knowledge
- engage directly with local communities in identifying needs, setting priorities and taking action
- develop 'joined up' approaches to tackle complex change issues.

Partnership working requires time and skills. Primary care personnel, and GPs in particular, have a rather poor reputation for partnership working on the whole within interdisciplinary and inter-sector working. This is something that needs to be addressed both within pre-registration and postgraduate training programmes. Some of the requirements for the development of 'healthy alliances' – partnerships for health improvement and collective change – are shown in Box 6.4.

Box 6.4: Characteristics of 'healthy alliances'[17]

- **Relationships**: an active and dynamic core group drawn from the partner agencies characterised by shared vision, a common agenda, agreed priorities, openness about self interest, mutual respect, trust.
- **Goals and targets**: shared understanding of the concept of health and inter-agency working's contribution to health gain, learning from and prioritising with local communities, leading to the establishment of broad goals and negotiated targets and commitment to a specific plan of action.
- **Activity**: beyond just the formal structures established by the alliance, development of informal networks, commitment and action throughout partner agencies and wider.
- **Shared resources**: in terms of core funding, time, information, political support 'in kind' contributions, resulting in shared balance of power based on inputs.
- **Community involvement**: wide range of approaches and activity demonstrated to ensure continuous dialogue with, and grounding in, local communities.
- **Co-ordination**: identifiable dedicated support drawing on a wide range of skills such as communication, negotiation, organisation and planning.
- **A capacity to learn**: learning by active experimentation and 'doing' and able to turn that learning to practical use.

Organisational development within primary care organisations

Organisational development is recognised by the Department of Health as an important dimension of community development.

'... organisation development, and a cultural shift, will be necessary if public service organisations are to build into their mainstream agenda the making of effective, equal partnerships with local people. Such change can only come about by building appropriate knowledge, skills, attitudes and relationships within organisations.'[18]

Detailed assessment and action planning tools to assist organisations in assessing their abilities to engage effectively with communities and plan their organisational change agendas are emerging. In Bradford, for example, a multi-agency team has developed a tool, piloted with two PCTs (*see* Box 6.5).

Box 6.5: 'How well are you doing on community involvement? A self-assessment tool for organisations'[19]

The indicators cover six key questions, each with a number of sub-questions:

1   Is the diversity of communities reflected in everything the organisation does?
2   Do the procedures in your organisation make it easy for communities to understand and participate?
3   Have you an effective communication strategy that meets the needs of all stakeholders?
4   Do you ensure that all the people involved in running your organisation have the knowledge, skills and support necessary to engage with the community?
5   Are all communities involved in the full range of decision making?
6   Do communities have any access to and control over resources?

Role of CD in delivering primary care

There are literally thousands of CD initiatives around the country which are delivering primary care – in relation to mental, physical, spiritual, emotional, social and economic well being. The following case example is used to highlight some of the effective work that is under way.

Case example: Community Health Project in Waltham Forest

The Community Health Project in Waltham Forest developed out of a partnership between the local Housing Action Trust (HAT), the health authority and local residents in 1994. It is now a NOF Healthy Living Centre managed by the Walthamstow, Leyton and Leytonstone PCT. One aspect was forging close links with local GPs, and setting up a referral system from

GPs to the various services and support that the project offers. Local people can also self refer to most of the services. In 1999, 90% of GPs in the borough were making referrals. The project has developed further through SRB finance and the NOF lottery fund and is now profiled.

Aims and early work

- To work with local people to improve access to services by piloting new models of care and/or facilitating access to existing services.
- To support and develop individual and community skills to enable local people to take more control of their health.
- To explore how existing services might better meet the needs of local people.
- To inform commissioning and partnership working.

Developing user-oriented service delivery

A rapid appraisal approach was used (*see* Chapter 3) to identify local needs and priorities, involving both local people and GPs. Mental health, back and skeletal problems and a range of health promotion issues were identified. As a result a number of services were developed which now operate directly from the project. These are as follows:

- **Counselling**: seven paid staff, working within three teams – generic/ outreach; older people and carers outreach; refugees and asylum seekers. A bursary scheme to provide training opportunities and placements for counsellors in specific local community languages is also in place as a response to locally identified needs.
- **A range of complementary therapies**: osteopathy; homoeopathy; aromatherapy; therapeutic massage; acupuncture: bursaries to enable local people to train and set up their own business in these disciplines are also offered.
- **Health Access Team**: a range of health clinics and outreach projects run by a team of five nurse and two sessional GPs and other health workers such as dietitians and chiropodists – offering open access/drop in clinics for confidential advice and then possibly referral on to appropriate services based in local community centres, sheltered housing schemes, schools, refugee centres, YMCA night shelter.
- **Specialist health access sessions**: female genital mutilation; refugees, asylum seekers and unaccompanied minors; homeless people.
- **Training and skilling programmes**: a range of health and personal development topics for local people, such as lay health worker skills; stress and anxiety management; TLC (Therapies for Lifestyle Changes); pain

management; health promotion and disease self management, e.g. diabetes.

- **Volunteer placement scheme**: for 20 volunteer counsellors.
- **Placements**: social work secondment, lay health workers and complementary therapy placements.
- **Salaried GP post**: to link to nurse led clinics, to work with homeless people and refugees and asylum seekers who have difficulty registering with local GPs.
- **Advocacy workers**: based in various drop-in centres and services.

From local project to wider strategic change and development

The project's ability to outreach to people and to respond to local needs meant it was able to set up substantial community representation on its early management structures. Users of specific services as well as other community residents became interested in getting involved alongside strong relationships with statutory, voluntary and independent sector organisations. Early success, the support of key individuals in partner agencies, and the developing vision of partner agencies, combined to allow the project not only to have a future as a local community initiative, but also to influence strategic thinking and planning across agencies.

Challenges for the project

The success of the project in securing major finance via NOF and SRB has had drawbacks. The team has expanded rapidly with 20 salaried staff, between 10 and 15 sessional paid staff and more than 20 regular volunteers, so the initial feel of a small community project has waned.

Although each service has maintained strong user involvement in both service planning and evaluation, community involvement in management has lapsed. Combined with the heavy internal management workload as a result of increased staff recruitment, and the detailed demands for regular statistical returns from funders, the emphasis shifted to a more inwardly focused 'alternative service delivery organisation'. There are now plans to re-establish a wider management structure, involving wider partners and a User and Community Board. More outreach and CD work is planned to complement the service delivery work.

Balancing out community development, service delivery and strategic partnership work has been a major challenge as the project has grown, and been buffeted by the external changes in the NHS. The demands of SRB and NOF for outcomes, most of which do not relate to CD criteria, have also been an added complexity. However, the project's basic philosophy and ethos have survived this period and the future for its CD work and ethos looks positive.

Conclusion

Community development and health work is not new, and much has been achieved over the last thirty years that has been visible as a distinct approach to health improvement and challenging inequalities. Emerging bodies, such as Patients' Forums and the Commission for Public and Patient Involvement, could provide much needed support and co-ordination. However, this is dependent on them adopting CD both as a key methodology, and underpinning values and principles.

Nevertheless, the current policy climate requires agencies to work in partnerships with local communities, and gives bodies like PCTs the lead responsibilities for tackling the complex range of factors that lead to health inequalities. This offers the exciting prospect that CD and health may move from their expression in short-term-funded initiatives to become a mainstream part of primary care practice.

References

1   Ashton J (1976) The Peckham Pioneer Health Centre: a reappraisal. *Community Health.* **8**: 132–7.

2   New Opportunities Fund (1999) *Healthy Living Centres: Information for Applicants, p. 7.* New Opportunities Fund, London.

3   NHS Executive Health Services Circular HSC 1198/065 9 April 1999. *The New NHS Modern and Dependable: establishing primary care groups.*

4   Fisher B and Gillam S (1999) Community development in the New NHS. *Br J Gen Pract.* **443**(49): 428–30.

5   Standing Conference for Community Development (2001) *Strategic Framework for Community Development.* SCCD, Sheffield.

6   Barr A and Hashagen S (2000) *ABCD Handbook: A framework for evaluating community development.* Community Development Foundation, London.

7   For example, see the first three chapters in Smithies J and Webster G (1998) *Community Involvement in Health: from passive recipients to active participants.* Ashgate Publishing, Aldershot.

8   The Scottish Office (1998) *Social Inclusion: opening the door to a better Scotland.* Scottish Office, Edinburgh.

9   Labonte R (1998) *A CD approach to Health Promotion: a background paper on practice tensions, strategic models and accountability requirements for health authority work on the broad determinants of health.* Health Education Board for Scotland and the Research Unit in Health and Behaviour Change, University of Edinburgh.

10   Freudenberg N (1997) *Health Promotion in the City.* Atlanta Center for Disease Control and Prevention.

11   Hashagen S (2000) *Developing Healthy Communities: achieving a consensus.* Discussion paper towards a conceptual framework for understanding the relationship between community development and health. Unpublished paper, available via the Scottish Community Development Centre. Tel: 01412481924.

12   NHS Executive (1998) *An organisational development resource for Primary Care Groups,* pp. 53–4. NHSE, Leeds.

13   NHS Executive (2000) *Primary Care Groups Public Engagement Toolkit.* NHS Executive Northern & Yorkshire, Durham.

14   Community Practitioners' and Health Visitors' Association: Community Development Special Interest Group. Website: www.msfcphva.org

15   Craig P (1996) Drumming up Health in Drumchapel: *Community Development Health Visiting.* **69**(11): 460–2.

16   Farrant W (1994) 'Health For All' in the inner city: exploring the implications for medical education. *Critical Public Health.* **5**(1): 22–31.

17   Powell M (1993) *Healthy Alliances.* King's Fund, London.

18   King's Fund Keypoints (2001) *What's to stop us? Overcoming barriers to public sector engagement with local communities.* Summary report of work commissioned by the Department of Health, London.

19   Fairfax P, South J, Green E *et al. Bradford Community Involvement Indicators Tool.* Forthcoming.

CHAPTER 7

Community Action on Health: marrying community development and primary care

Philip Crowley and Debbie Freake

Introduction

Previous chapters have discussed community-oriented approaches to health (*see* Chapter 4) and the principles and practice of community development (*see* Chapter 6). Both have highlighted the potential and considerable challenges of marrying these with primary care. This chapter tells of a community development, Community Action on Health, that has built partnerships between primary care organisations and local communities in Newcastle upon Tyne. Community Action on Health has been funded through primary care in Newcastle upon Tyne since 1995, receiving an NHS Equality Award in 1998 for tackling health inequalities. There is a particular focus on working with groups of identity and interest that frequently experience discrimination.

Policy context

Partnership and accountability, alongside user and patient participation in deliberations about health and health services are firmly on the agenda.[1–5] Their implementation[6] and the systematic collection of user and carer views and experiences in assessing NHS performance are regarded as vital.[7]

The *NHS Plan*[2] and *Shifting the Balance of Power within the NHS*[3] promise to shift power and resources not only to front-line staff but also to the people who use and pay for the service. Indeed the Health and Social Care Act, 2001[8] places a new duty on the NHS to consult and involve patients and the public in decision making.

Consumer versus democratic accountability

Latest policy seeks to ensure that wider public involvement and the concept of 'community voice' are adopted, in particular to tackle health inequalities.[9,10] However, recent policy also commits the NHS to a more consumerist style despite attempting democratic accountability through 'Overview and Scrutiny Committees', and encouraging wider involvement through 'local networks'.

The role for primary care trust (PCT) Patients' Forums risks losing the wider community agenda by focusing solely on a health *service* agenda (involving patients in designing NHS care) to the exclusion of marginalised groups that a community development approach seeks to engage (working with citizens and communities to improve health and influence healthcare).[11] Although commitment to comprehensive involvement and minimum standards is welcome, the difficulties of enabling community participation through a 'one-size-fits-all' centrally imposed model are of concern.

Primary care and communities

As Chapters 4 and 6 have noted, progress toward primary care decision making that involves users and carers or the wider community has been slow.[12–15] There have been some notable exceptions[16] but few managers have experience or understanding of public involvement.[17] Even where there is commitment, participation by local people is thought difficult to achieve.[18]

The emergence of Primary Care Groups (PCGs) in April 1999 enabled groups of GP practices and staff working together to develop services in geographical areas rather than focus exclusively on their own practice patients. Their transformation in 2002 to PCTs and care trusts, often co-terminous with local authorities whose role in health has been promoted by government, anticipates greater partnership working on health determinants.

Newcastle West

Newcastle West PCG, where the Community Action on Health project started in 1995, covered a population of 114 000, including a significant black and ethnic minority population.[19] There is high morbidity and mortality with evidence of differential access to healthcare provision in comparison with other localities in the district.[20] One third of all children were born into poverty and there were high unemployment and levels of low paid work. On average, death before the age of 65 was almost twice as likely in the West City than the rest of the North East region.

Early History of Community Action on Health

Locality commissioning

In the early 1990s a review of health services in Newcastle threatened the future of the district general hospital at the heart of the socio-economically disadvantaged inner west of Newcastle. This was a major employer of local people, favoured by local general practitioners above the nearby central teaching hospital. The threat to the hospital galvanised local primary healthcare workers into collective action.

A group of general practitioners, many of whom were opposed to fund-holding, formed across practices to look at various models of collective commissioning. In response, the health authority divided the entire district into localities. Each locality appointed a GP adviser to work with the health authority, and each was allocated a small budget to be used in helping to address the specific health needs of that locality.

First steps

In order to decide on the best use of these development funds, the Inner West Locality GP Group commissioned an appraisal of health needs in 1995. This sought the views of local people and primary healthcare workers, including the voluntary sector. A worker (PC) was employed for a six-month period and visited all the primary care teams, local health service management and over 90 community groups.

This led to a community conference, attended by some 150 people, which identified priority areas shared by local people and workers alike – young people, mental health, excluded families, older people and black and ethnic minorities.[21]

From local appraisal to community accountability

The community called for the opportunity for ongoing involvement, with a dedicated worker and a commitment to transparency and continuous dialogue. The locality commissioning group and the health authority funded a full time community development worker for the locality who was accountable to the local community and independent of health service management. This was considered vital to the success of the work.[22]

The locality commissioning group prioritised the areas defined by the initial appraisal of local health needs. As the priorities were based on broad client groups rather than services, the locality group was encouraged to adopt a less medically-focused model of health than that used in neighbouring localities to develop primary care. Where groups formed to undertake new areas of work, their make-up reflected this more social model of health including community representatives as well as health and social care workers, in statutory and voluntary sectors.

Community Action on Health

The values and practice of community development are considered in some detail in Chapter 5. The Community Action on Health (CAH) project has used a community development approach to realise community participation in health issues.[23] This seeks to go beyond consultation and needs assessment in trying to develop local communities to act on their own health agendas. A clear commitment to equity and challenging discrimination informs the work.

The initial worker has visited over 90 local groups each year and prepared an annual report from the issues raised. The annual Community Conference on Health, attended by over 200 people, determines the priorities for the following year's work. An action plan is then taken forward by the worker, steered by the CAH committee of local residents, who are nominated by the local community groups.

The CAH committee elected two representatives (sharing one vote) onto the board of the (now) Newcastle PCT in place of the usual lay representative. They followed up the issues raised with an action plan and gave direction to the work of the development worker – this was the prime method for accountability of the worker to the local community.

CAH work focuses on networking and bringing together groups around common issues with the relevant health services and local authority management to push for the changes the community identified as a priority. The work has actively sought to involve groups who are often particularly marginalised such as black and ethnic minority communities, lesbian and gay groups, older people, adolescents and people with a physical and sensory disability.[24] In some cases this has had clear resource implications, for instance the need to provide sign language interpreters for deaf people.

Stimulation of change

A number of new services have resulted from the CAH work, demonstrating a clear response to community priorities and an understanding of the social model of health. Many initiatives, because of community involvement, attracted new funds to the health service from joint finance and regeneration funds. The examples below illustrate the willingness of the early primary care commissioning group to provide different models of community services and, importantly, services which were not necessarily provided within a traditional general practice setting.

Younger people

An inter-agency youth strategy group formed which successfully secured SRB funding for a dedicated facility for young people. The resultant Youth Enquiry Service provides information, counselling and advice to young people on a range of issues including sexual health, drugs and alcohol, employment, housing and benefits in a youth base.

Young families

Work by the community development worker with local parent and toddler groups and tenants' organisations highlighted the isolation and vulnerability of some families, especially those who had just moved into the area. Families First, funded through the original primary care locality budget, was developed in partnership with other local family support initiatives.

This provides peer support to vulnerable and isolated families. The model was developed by a multi-agency group in preference to the more obvious approach of employing additional nursery nurses. Working in partnership with NCH Action for Children, the initiative employed and trained local parents to provide support, and involve users in the management of the service.

South Asian communities

The community development work with local ethnic minority groups contributed to the development of a dedicated counselling service based in the community and outside of general practice.

Case example: Access for the deaf community to the local acute NHS trust

At the annual community conference local representatives of the deaf community highlighted problems experienced in accessing services in the local acute trust. Incorporated into the conference report this became a priority for action in the following year. A meeting was arranged with the local deaf centre and it was decided to invite members of the deaf community to the centre to discuss their health needs with management representatives from the main trusts.

An evening meeting was held at their usual venue and conducted through British Sign Language with interpretation for the managers. Fundamental problems were identified including the absence of any minicoms in the trust buildings. A series of meetings between representatives of the deaf community and trust management followed.

Eventually the trust agreed to install minicoms in all key access points and to make mobile minicoms available to inpatients. Deaf awareness days were organised and an advisory group, operational to this day, was established with representation from organisations of disabled people.

Developing PCG and PCT with Community Action on Health

The ability to consider the locality as more than a cluster of general practices and their registered patients allowed the Locality Commissioning Group to develop rapidly as an organisation committed to partnership. Although the early Locality Commissioning Group was initially dominated by GPs, a multi-disciplinary, multi-agency implementation group developed with community involvement, which allowed for wider ownership of the work.

Growth of Primary Care Group

As the Inner West Locality expanded to become a pilot PCG, as part of the National GP Commissioning Pilot the group was well placed to define a board structure that was balanced in terms of stakeholder input. Local GPs declined the opportunity to take a majority position on the PCG board, and initial professional defensiveness on all sides rapidly gave way to constructive partnership working.

Co-opted community development workers supporting additional lay members were universally accepted as a constructive addition, and 'Community Concerns' still remains a standing PCT agenda item today.

Initially mirroring the model of Community Action on Health, the various PCG stakeholders met in their respective professional groups. Interestingly, whilst the other groups flourished the GP forum withered. Given the extensive GP involvement in PCG work it is hard to interpret this as apathy or cynicism, and appeared more to reflect the confidence of local GPs in PCG mechanisms and their ability to ensure their views and interests were adequately represented.

Mutuality

The development of the Locality Commissioning Group that became Newcastle West Primary Care Group occurred simultaneously with that of the Community Action on Health project. It is perhaps this concurrent growth which helped to foster the excellent relationship between the two.

The Locality Commissioning Group and subsequently the PCG were evolving organisations upon which a fledgling Community Action on Health tried to make an impression. Both organisations were initially dependent on a few key individuals who communicated closely and learnt together, developing early trust and mutual respect.

The PCG struggled to meet the need for their members to participate fully in the health and regeneration agenda in West Newcastle because of the considerable clinical workload for the primary care professionals in general practice. Despite this, the enthusiasm and commitment of coalface workers in primary care have been remarkable, and have enabled delivery of a complex and ambitious business plan.

Community participation in Newcastle PCT

Inspired by the model, the other two local PCGs in Newcastle sought to develop their own 'brand' of Community Action on Health. In April 2001 as the PCGs in Newcastle joined to form a single primary care trust, Community Action on Health also developed into a city-wide network.

The three projects now come together under the umbrella of Community Action on Health Newcastle. There is currently a network of ongoing, supported, community involvement initiatives, broadly based around the three locality (previous PCG) areas across Newcastle, entirely funded by the PCT.

Newcastle Health Partnership

The Newcastle Health Partnership (a partnership between the health authority, local authority, NHS and primary care trust, voluntary sector, community and universities and now a subset of the newer Local Strategic Partnership) adopted a strategy for community participation.

Based on community development principles this has enabled the funding of a city-wide co-ordination post to create links between the different community development initiatives funded by the PCT and to ensure the involvement of communities of interest in an emerging city-wide community action group. Links have been created between the communities of different districts in the Tyne and Wear Health Action Zone and 'Real Voices' conferences have been organised to bring together communities from across the area and to establish their agenda.

Evaluation of Community Action on Health

An independent evaluation of the CAH work in 1999 found its community development approach had been effective in engaging with a large number of local community groups and representatives. Moreover, this had created a systematic focus for what was then the West PCG on health inequalities and discrimination against minority groups.

Professional perceptions

Professionals were shown to appreciate the project for its awareness raising of minority group issues. Most felt that it was a good use of health service money, leading to better identification of needs and more appropriate services, and introducing an element of accountability into health service delivery.[25]

Community impact

Community representatives felt that it had helped them better understand the issues of discrimination against minority groups in that it was the first time some of them had worked with disabled or black groups. Through its annual round of visits to 84 community groups (the main method of identifying local issues) the project was estimated to be in direct contact with over 1200 local people (numbers were counted at meetings).

Community representation

A criticism commonly levelled at community involvement exercises is that they attract the same group of 'professional meeting-attenders' or establish a self-sustaining clique, which is unrepresentative of the wider community. The evaluation has shown that Community Action on Health has developed a more inclusive process, which strengthens the links between community activists and the wider community. This allows a more accountable and 'networked' representation than is likely solely through appointed lay representatives on a primary care group board or non-executive primary care trust board members.

At the time of writing, a further evaluation has found that local health service managers maintain that the work of Community Action on Health has influenced the way decisions are made in Newcastle. Local black workers see tackling racial discrimination as one of the key strengths of the project's work.

Challenges for the project

Evaluation highlights a number of challenges for the project.

- As it is a networking project it relies on the strength of local community activity. This way of working can be problematic in areas where there is little collective community activity.
- The workers in the project can spend a lot of time in meetings with the statutory agencies and this can detract from the local development work

with communities. Getting the right balance between these two arms of the project's work is a challenge.

- There is a risk that the project workers may be drawn into speaking *on behalf of* the community in meetings, thus excluding community representatives.
- The project may be seen as the sole conduit for local community participation, marginalising other valid community initiatives.
- There is a clear necessity to balance the need to challenge the system with the need to develop work in co-operation with it. There is a danger of CAH workers becoming too cosy with those who represent the statutory agencies.
- CAH and other successful community involvement initiatives need to carefully consider how they will relate to new national structures for patient and public involvement. There is a danger that unless integration or co-operation are ensured, existing successful work will be undermined or effort unnecessarily duplicated with resultant 'involvement fatigue'. In particular the approach to a PCT Patient Forum requires considerable thought.

Conclusion

This chapter has described a community development approach to building a partnership between a PCT and the local communities it serves. The project has demonstrated that this approach is sustainable if funding is stable – it has remained vibrant and productive for over seven years.

The project has demonstrated the importance of engaging local communities on their own agenda and of ensuring the participation of marginalised and minority groups who are typically excluded from most community participation initiatives in health.

Key messages

- Community development can engage local communities in tackling health inequalities and overcoming barriers to service access for minority groups.
- Community development skills and experience are critical.
- Sustainability requires clear feedback to local communities and demonstrable progress on community concerns.
- Any community development post needs to be accountable to the local community and independent of the primary care trust and health service management.

- Primary care trust boards should ensure direct supported community input beyond the contribution of non-executive board members. The role of the new Patient Forums requires careful consideration.
- The current focus on patients and PFs should not divert attention from greater efforts that attempt to democratise health service decision making and develop local communities.

References

1   Department of Health (1997) *The New NHS: Modern, dependable*. HMSO, London.

2   Department of Health (2000) *The NHS Plan. A plan for investment, a plan for reform*. HMSO, London.

3   Department of Health (2001) *Shifting the Balance of Power within the NHS*. HMSO, London.

4   Department of Health (2001) *Involving Patients and the Public in Healthcare*. A Discussion Document. HMSO, London.

5   Department of Health (2002) *Involving Patients and the Public in Healthcare: Response to the listening exercise*. HMSO, London.

6   NHS Executive (1998) *The New NHS: modern, dependable*. Health Services Circular 139.

7   NHS Executive (1998) *A First Class Service: quality in the new NHS*. Department of Health, London.

8   Health and Social Care Act (2001) C.15. HMSO, London.

9   Fisher B, Neve H and Heritage Z (1999) Community development, user involvement and primary healthcare. *BMJ*. **318**: 749–50.

10   Department of Health (1998) *Saving Lives: Our healthier nation*. HMSO, London.

11   Hansard (2002) NHS Reform in Health Care Professions Bill. Hansard, House of Lords. Vol 636. 13 June 2002.

12   Regen E, Smith J and Shapiro J (1998) *First off the Starting Block: Lessons from GP commissioning pilots for primary care groups*. Health Services Management Centre, University of Birmingham, Birmingham.

13   Coote A (1993) Public participation in decisions about health care. *Critical Public Health*. **4**: 36–49.

14   Freeman R, Gillam S, Shearin C, *et al*. *Community Development and Involvement in Primary Care*, VII. King's Fund, London.

15   Smithies J and Webster G (1998) *Community Involvement in Health – from passive recipients to active participants*. Ashgate, Aldershot.

16   O'Keefe E and Hogg C (1999) Public participation and marginalised groups: the community development model. *Health Expectations*. **2**(4): 245–54.

17 Lupton C, Peckham S and Taylor P (1998) *Managing Public Involvement in Healthcare Purchasing*. Open University Press, Buckingham.

18 Taylor P, Peckham S and Turton P (1998) A Public Health Model of Primary Care – from concept to reality. Public Health Alliance, Birmingham.

19 Freake D, Crowley P, Steiner M, *et al.* (1997) Local heroes. *Health Services Journal*, 10 July: 28–9.

20 Directorate of Public Health (1997) *Health Profiles by Locality* (2). Newcastle and North Tyneside Health Authority, Newcastle.

21 Crowley P (1995) *Health and health care in the West End of Newcastle*: A report of a rapid appraisal and the proceedings of a workshop to discuss health needs in the Inner West of Newcastle. Newcastle and North Tyneside Health Authority, Newcastle.

22 Zutshi M (1990) Community development from within a statutory setting – a contradiction in terms? In: *Roots and Branches*. OU/HEA Winter School on Community Development and Health, London.

23 Standing Conference for Community Development (1992) *Working Statement on Community Development*. SCCD, Sheffield.

24 Crowley P (1998) *Community Action on Health Annual Report*. Community Action on Health, Newcastle.

25 Green J (1999) *Community Action on Health*. Social Welfare Research Unit, University of Northumbria at Newcastle.

CHAPTER 8

Sure Start, making a difference? A parent's perspective

Sandra Wathall

'The aim of Sure Start is to work with parents, parents-to-be and children to promote the physical, intellectual and social development of babies and young children – particularly those who are disadvantaged – so that they can flourish at home and when they get to school, and thereby break the cycle of disadvantage for the current generation of young children.'

Sure Start Unit

Introduction

I got involved in Sure Start as a local parent with a young son. I find the whole ethos of Sure Start really exciting. It represents an incredible shift in public thinking from problem tackling to problem prevention. I believe for the first time, that the government is taking on board what therapists, teachers and social workers have perhaps known all along, that what happens in childhood has lasting effects on an individual and that disadvantage in childhood can create dysfunctional adults.

The grand plan is to eradicate child poverty within twenty years and break the cycle of disadvantage as it runs through generations. What is exciting is that the government is putting money into the community to do this, not dictating how it should be done but empowering communities to create for themselves. So all Sure Start programmes are individually tailored to meet the needs of the neighbourhood in which they are housed. This means local people are consulted and engaged in the process.

Sure Start in Birmingham

Sixty Sure Start programmes were launched in 1999. Birmingham was one of the 'trailblazers'. There are now ten programmes in Birmingham alone with two more in the pipeline and 364 currently nationwide. There is a plan for a total of 502 by 2004.

Areas are selected on the basis of 'deprivation', however our project in Billesley, an outer ring estate in Birmingham, was selected as a trailblazer because it already had an established Children and Parents' Centre, providing some of the services Sure Start advocated – mum and toddler groups, pre-school playgroup and so on. There was seen to be a natural community who made use of existing facilities, so the boundary was drawn to include no more than 1000 children in the 0–4 age range and roads that were within pram-pushing distance of the Centre.

On motherhood

Sure Start arrived on my doorstep when my little boy was two years old. I had moved into the area just before getting pregnant and was relatively new to Birmingham, so I had few connections and little support. I had chosen to be a stay-at-home mum, believing I was the best person to care for my baby, but it was hard going and I found myself battling with despair.

Nothing can prepare you for motherhood. No amount of reading or attendance at ante-natal groups can quite illustrate the impact of all those physical and emotional demands twenty-four hours a day, seven days a week. There is no switching off.

I came to it all late. I was 37, newly married and deposited in a new area with no family or friends close at hand to call upon. My husband was very supportive and fortunate enough to work flexi-time, but for the most part I was on my own with this little baby who totally depended upon me.

I had my son by caesarean section, which wasn't the best start for either of us. Although I had been conscious, I had not seen or felt my son being born. It took me many weeks to adjust and accept that he was mine. I felt someone could have brought him in from another room. Thankfully, my determination to breastfeed helped us bond, despite it being toe-curlingly painful.

Seeking connections

Fortunately, there was a breastfeeding group which I attended, but at that time it only ran once a month and not being a driver getting there involved catching two buses. I tried other mother and baby groups but everything felt like an effort. The first six weeks when I really needed support and contact, there was nothing. Eventually, when my son was six weeks old, I was able to join a group at the local health centre. It was such a relief, something local that I could walk to.

There always seemed to be this big assumption that having a baby gives you lots in common with other women. It **doesn't**. Sitting around, sleep-deprived and in shock, feeling and looking like zombies, with no shared history, feeling like there's no future, just endless need, twenty-four hours a day, every day, for ever. What had I done?

Running the gamut of emotion

I have a good husband. He didn't work long hours, or go out regularly in the evenings, he was always at the end of the 'phone if I needed him and would come home early when the stress in my voice demanded it. But I couldn't tell him how I really felt. The sense of bleakness, how I fantasised about running away, getting on a train or just walking, or worse still....

A woman I had made friends with at an ante-natal class suffered from debilitating post-natal depression. I didn't think it applied to me, after all this was a very much wanted baby and he was so beautiful and healthy, I should have been on top of the world. Thank goodness my health visitor encouraged me to attend a group she was running. There, for the first time I could sit and talk whilst my son was cared for elsewhere in a crèche. I could have my needs back and finally express out loud the level of my despair and the shame that went with it.

Getting involved in Sure Start

When my son was about a year old we moved on from our weekly group at the health centre, to a group at the Children and Parents' Centre, which was ultimately to become the centre for the Sure Start Programme. The head of the Centre was very good about consulting users of the facilities and I guess this is where the initial plans were laid down for Sure Start.

I felt so grateful for the facilities and the support of the staff that I wanted to give something back. An advisory board was being formed to oversee the Sure Start Programme and needed a percentage of local parents so, with encouragement, I agreed to stand and was duly elected, not knowing quite what I could contribute. I had been out of the world of work for some time and felt rather intimidated by all the smart suits I encountered at the initial meetings. But I persisted, helped I suspect by my role as secretary. At the first meeting it was announced that the parents would be expected to take on roles within the board, much to our horror. It is interesting to note, however, that the ones who adopted roles are the ones who have stuck with it.

I don't imagine it was easy for the professionals to meet each other, never mind with the presence of lay people. It always struck me as very formal and very 'male' for what was essentially a meeting of women – of the twenty or so members only two were men. It also wasn't inclusive, assumptions were made about knowledge, jargon bandied around. This was not exactly empowering for the under confident.

What made it work for me was the support of one or two key people I could call on for 'translation' and the fact that free childcare was provided – there was a crèche on site. That same year I became involved with a group to develop a local newsletter for Sure Start. I enjoyed being a part of what was going on, meeting other people where I could be more than just a mum.

Peer consultation: exploring needs

In order to find out what facilities were needed by local people, a survey was conducted using local parents as interviewers. I also became involved with this. It created temporary employment and proved valuable as a confidence booster. We got a fascinating insight into what was available in the area and what was perceived to be available.

One of the biggest messages from parents was that there was not enough information about what was available in terms of provision. People were not aware of the range of facilities for young children nor the difference between them, e.g. stay and play or mum and toddler groups, playgroup or pre-school. However, there was perceived to be a need for more parent and toddler groups, for crèche facilities, 'somewhere to leave the children whilst I go shopping', for playgroups and holiday provision, plus a desire for a central source of information.

There also appeared to be a particular gap in provision for children between the ages of 18 months and 2½ years, a time when many parents felt it was most needed as their children were becoming more sociable. It was discovered that, of the people interviewed, over 20% of families with a child under 3 were not using any form of childcare or educational provision or attending any groups. Parents of children with special needs commented that it was often not until their children got to school that they received any support or felt they were heard. It was discovered that, for many people, getting into the first provision, getting a foot on the ladder as it were, was incredibly important as a means of gaining information about other facilities.

More local research followed with local parents trained and facilitated as interviewers. This looked at the quality of life of those living in the area and hopes and expectations for them and their families. Parents generally wanted their children to have a better educational chance and to achieve more than they were able to themselves, to be healthy and to lead a life marked by integration and acceptance. There were also important messages about themselves – they sought greater recognition as parents, while for others greater flexible support and childcare to get back into work or further education were important.

What has involvement meant for me?

I found it hard to understand why other parents did not want to get involved. On various occasions I have felt I am the token parent. Is it because people already feel too much is being asked of them in looking after their families, holding down a job, just getting through? Is it because people feel they have nothing to contribute?

I cannot make claims for my own contribution, that is for others to assess. What I do know and am just beginning to grasp, is the very real difference that involvement has made to my life. For starters, having a break from my child, from the intensity of that one-to-one relationship so that I could focus on other things; mental stimulation; being around active members of the community and people who are good at what they do; absorbing a sense of excellence.

Building confidence and self-belief, developing new skills, like recording minutes and remembering old ones (I did have a life before I became a mum!). On top of all this, a sense of service to my community, having been a nomad all my adult life. I had never had any previous commitment to the area in which I was living. This has given me a sense of belonging, which I value. I have also been fortunate enough to be privy to a lot of information that other local parents haven't due to my involvement, so I know about some of the ongoing challenges.

Lots to sort out

The Children and Parents' Centre has been redeveloped to accommodate the expanding services and team. Whilst this was happening, the Sure Start staff were housed in temporary offices at a local church, which has not exactly helped cohesion. The Sure Start programme and the Children and Parents' project have had different and separate management structures, with an overlap of a few personnel, which we are now attempting to merge. Each also has its own funding arrangement, the Children and Parents' Centre being a voluntary organisation. So, lots to sort out. There has also been the ongoing problem of staff changes; given only short contracts with fear of non-renewal of funds, people move on and maybe this kind of working isn't for everyone.

Bottom up 'at the front line'

Sure Start is different because of its bottom up rather than top down approach. It is about involving local parents and local practitioners in the decision making and planning for their community at ground level, rather than having someone dictate from on high about what is needed and where money should be spent. It involves a more holistic approach to problems, encouraging the breakdown of barriers between different professions, utilising the resources of various agencies that share a common purpose in dealing with families and young children and getting them to work together.

The emphasis is on empowering parents, building confidence and self-esteem to enable them to do the best for their children. It does this in very practical ways. For example, by setting up parent and toddler groups and showing parents the kind of play they can experiment with at home, using very simple, everyday material. One of the targets for Sure Start Programmes is that all children under four in their catchment area must have access to high quality play and learning opportunities.

Making a difference?

An evaluation of the programme is currently under way, so it will be interesting to see how the community views the impact of Sure Start. Certainly, many people will be making far more use of facilities than ever before. The new building is stretched to capacity running new mum and toddler groups; it has extended its pre-school provision, has created ante-natal groups run by a midwife and a parent support worker and it now has trained inclusion workers working with families of children with special needs.

Then there is a whole army of outreach workers who go out into the community. Every family with a new baby or a child under four is contacted and consulted regarding their views and needs and given information about facilities and groups. For families experiencing crisis, there are trained volunteers offering practical support within the home.

A toy library has been created in a local school, providing good quality equipment and play material for a nominal fee. There are small grants available to fund local projects and Sure Start have provided backing for the development of a local business, Fun on the Run, a mobile crèche run by and for the community. So, it is not hard to see evidence. So much has changed.

Sadly, some of these services arrived a little late for me and many of the people whose input and suggestions helped create them. But at least we were able to draw on our experience, which was seen as valid, and make a difference for others. We have helped create a more localised system that supports parents from the beginning, even before their child is born, educating, enlightening, empowering; supporting them to do their best so that their children have a good start in life.

We need to start now

The government talks about 'long-termism' and wants the programmes to be sustainable, but the money will begin to tail off. So, then there is talk of mainstreaming, which I suppose means taking what we have learnt and making it common practice. And why not? This is radical. This is saying that people matter, that children matter, that how we raise our children affects the whole society we live in. If we really care about making a difference for future generations we have to start early. We need to start now.

CHAPTER 9

The Flower 125 Health Club

Bethan Plant and Siobhan McFeely

'On Wenday the group was all toking abut all of overy hersyns we aur dowing a very los of stuf we aur all aur injouing it – it will be fun of all the stuth.'

'On Wednesday the group was all talking about all of ourselves, we are doing a very lot of stuff, we are all enjoying it. It will be fun all of the stuff.'

A 13-year-old girl participating in a Flower 125 Health Workshop

Introduction

The Flower 125 Health Club is a multi-agency initiative for young people. It aims to improve the health profile of local young people, to raise confidence and self-esteem and to help these individuals to develop an increased knowledge about health. This needs to be done, and in new and innovative ways.

Established in March 1998 the project initially involved a health promotion specialist, a practice nurse, a learning mentor, and an independent drama facilitator. Staff from different organisations developed a twenty-week programme of workshops, which look at a variety of health related issues. These are then explored through drama. At the end of the twenty weeks a drama production is presented to the young people's peers, thus introducing an element of peer education.

Starting points as a practice nurse

Siobhan McFeely
This type of work was *very* new to my role as a nurse. Having worked in general practice for over ten years and as a nurse for over twenty years, the

thought of starting to work with vulnerable young people was daunting. The traditional way of working was to see patients in surgery, or to visit them at home, and to deliver care to 'sick' patients. Health education may happen, opportunistically, as the need or situation arises.

Having recently completed a Bachelor's degree I was keen to apply my new found knowledge. This project grew out of a meeting with a health promotion specialist. I talked about how I felt that young people didn't seem to access healthcare in surgery and thus the chance for health education was lost. This new work was to challenge my whole philosophy.

The health promotion specialist

Bethan Plant

My role as a health promotion specialist involved working with primary care staff in developing joint work within the local community. Having experience of setting up and establishing multi-agency initiatives I was eager to work with the practice nurse in developing a project on a local estate.

As a qualified youth worker I am aware of the health needs of young people. Many young people do not access healthcare services or find they do not meet their needs. Many are concerned about confidentiality,[1] being particularly worried that they may be seen by other family members in the doctor's surgery. Often young people find consulting times inconvenient and think that primary care doesn't know how to work with them – services are not 'young people friendly'.

Young people and health: tackling inequalities

In the new agenda for tackling health and inequalities, partnership at a local level is seen as the key to success in improving health.[2] The emphasis for the '125 Health Project' is on joint working so that it meets young people's needs at a local level. The work of the 125 Flower Estate Project speaks to government priorities such as reducing the uptake of smoking among young people,[3] tackling the underlying causes of teenage pregnancy,[4] providing better education about sexual health and relationships and addressing young people's mental health and improving their self-esteem.

There has not been enough emphasis on prevention, and services have been poorly designed to meet the real circumstances of the poorest young people. Services have also failed to adapt to new problems experienced by young people such as poor mental health, substance misuse and challenging behaviour.[5] The 125 Health Project focuses on addressing vulnerable young people's needs. It works with the most hard to reach young people and attempts to tackle new problems that young people are experiencing.

The local context

The estate on which the project was first run is recognised as an area of poverty with a high number of young people under the age of eighteen living in households with no earners. The estate also has a high rate of crime. It has been through several periods of transition, with numerous new families moving onto the estate and then quickly moving away. There was talk of part of the estate being demolished and families being relocated. Many of the young people have extended families spanning three generations, born and bred locally. The estate was unsettled with the prospect of the possible upheaval.

> 'It's horrible, have you seen the houses? ... everyone walks round looking dead miserable. It's crap ... we've got a right bad name.'

Life on the estate was not easy, and young people knew the reputation that the estate had.

> '... twocking – nicking cars and loads of people round here are in prison. People have even got killed, it's rough. It worries me we get called bad things.'

Getting started

In order to secure staff time, a proposal for an initial six-month project was drawn up. This set out the evidence for why such a project was needed and was based on data collected from a variety of sources,[6] local council reports,[7] and information from the local GP practice where the practice nurse worked. This helped to build up a profile of the area and also to look at the provisions for young people locally – of which there were none!

It was felt that workshops would be more appropriate to raise and address health issues here. We started with a great deal of enthusiasm but failed at the first post. Many of the young people were known to the practice nurse, and it was important not to let their reputation influence it negatively. The initial session whilst planned and well attended, did not achieve what was intended. Our main problem was disruptive and violent behaviour. After major problems (being threatened with a gate no longer on its hinges) it was soon time to re-evaluate.

The options were to stop the work or find a new way of working. Having suffered an enormous amount of stress and trauma, the first option was the most attractive. A great deal of thought went into our decision. The over-riding feeling was that if we gave up we would be compounding a pattern that many of these young people were repeatedly subjected to. We could have given up and failed. We decided to stop to reflect and then resume with a different tack.

Second chance saloon

We revisited our original project proposal. Although we felt we had prepared well, we had failed to take into account the poor literacy of the young people involved, their behaviour and how we could maintain their concentration over a period of time. We needed to look at a new way of recruiting young people to attend the project. Previously, young people had been recruited through school assemblies and via posters distributed in schools and posted into houses on the estate. Clearly, the young people needed more information about the project and we needed to have contact with the young people's parents as well.

Developing links with two youth workers on the estate proved to be invaluable, as they had good relationships with the young people. Through our links we were able to target the project at those young people who the youth workers felt would benefit most. These were young people who lived on the estate, many of whom did not regularly attend school or who were often temporarily excluded.

The project team, now with the two youth workers, visited each young person's home and met with the individual's parents. At this meeting each parent was given information about the project and asked to sign a parental consent form. It also provided an opportunity for the parents or young person to ask any questions. Making these home visits was crucial to the project work. This changed the atmosphere in the workshops. It was as though the young people felt that the staff were really committed to them because we had made the effort to actually go into their homes. In addition, a drama element was introduced to the workshops with a drama facilitator recruited to work with the young people to help address lack of concentration and improve behaviour.

The Flower 125 Club

The project runs for twenty weeks and involves up to fifteen young people aged 11–16 years participating in workshops focused on different health issues. Alternate weeks would be spent using drama as a vehicle to explore some of the issues raised during the health session. The work is based on a model, initially devised for working with children aged 3–8 years, developed by Caroline Webster Stratton.[8]

The young people involved

Young people living on the estate have low levels of self-esteem and are often in trouble at home or in school. Very rarely are they given any encouragement or praise. They openly admit that their behaviour is a problem.

> 'We are all dead mouthy and a bit rough – but no one is ever nice to us. At least if we kick off we get some attention then.'

Using a behavioural model

Expecting a child to function without praise or reward is unrealistic. The only way a child learns to engage in a particular behaviour is to have that behaviour reinforced.[8] The project gives young people praise but ignores any inappropriate behaviour. The young people only get attention if they are seen to be behaving appropriately.

Tangible rewards were used to support the model such as small items of toiletries, stickers, and pens. Often the young people themselves would decide who had worked the hardest and who deserved the reward at the end of each workshop. The young people were praised if they sat quietly, listened, contributed, worked hard and supported each other in the group. We simply offered praise for basic things such as sitting still or listening. In addition if someone received acknowledgement for their good behaviour they would be given an icon. The icon was a visual representation of the good behaviour.

Ignoring inappropriate behaviour was one of the most difficult techniques that we had to carry out. Teasing, arguing, swearing and being disruptive can be eliminated if they are systematically ignored. Staff avoided eye contact with the individual, we would physically move away from the young person but not leave the room, as soon as the behaviour stopped we would return our attention to the individual and staff would limit the amount of bad behaviour ignored.

This behavioural model had a huge impact on young people's behaviour. They themselves noticed a change.

> 'Things are better now – we are more good, we concentrate more and most of the time we sit down.'

Young people recognised what the staff were doing and the group began using the model on their own. We would find that the young people praised each other. If someone was behaving inappropriately the young people themselves would deal with the situation and encourage the individual to apologise and participate in the session.

> 'It's best when we work like this with icons an' stuff – cos if someone kicks off we calm 'em down. All us lot sort it out now – we do it together.'

The workshops in practice

All the workshops were planned and structured using the above model. The initial group of fifteen was too large to work with so we split this into two with different team names.

The very first workshop was used to provide the young people with an overview of the project. It started with all the staff introducing themselves and an ice breaker game was used. It was explained that we expected the young people to commit to the whole twenty weeks. The session moved on to explain and talk about what confidentiality meant so that the young people were aware of the issue from the start. Following on, the young people then devised and set their own ground rules.

Allowing the young people to devise the ground rules themselves encouraged the group to work together and discuss what they agreed to be acceptable. The ground rules were owned by them and when staff referred back to them the young people were reminded that they themselves had agreed them. At this session every young person also signed a 'contract'. This outlines to the young people their responsibility for their own behaviour.

The workshops used lots of 'hands on' activities. For example, during one session on alcohol we aimed to explore the effects of alcohol from different perspectives. The first activity started with the young people drawing round a group member. The outline of the body was then used to document the following:

- immediate effects of alcohol
- long-term effects of alcohol.

Once identified the group discussed if they felt they were positive or negative effects and why they felt this. The exercise raised a lot of discussion and was not only about their own 'lived experience' of alcohol. Various episodes of observing adults being drunk and behaving badly were recounted.

Role play was used to act out several scenarios, looking at possible outcomes in each of the situations. Spontaneous discussion was able to arise out of a trusting relationship with the project staff. This enabled the young people to talk about the issues they were faced with each day, and to look at alternatives in a positive and secure environment.

> '... we come and talk to ya – ya like second mums! ... 'cos you can say things in confidence and it dunt get out – I trust all you lot.'

During the whole of this session the young people were focused and well behaved. The session appeared to have 'real' meaning for them, they could understand and relate to the subject and, more importantly, contribute to the discussion. They knew that they were 'heard' and listened to, and for some of the young people the session appeared to have a profound effect or was cathartic.

Using drama

Drama was used to help explore some of the issues raised in the workshops. The drama facilitator worked with the young people to develop a short drama production. The young people performed the drama production to their peers in two different youth clubs. The overall principle is to raise the self-esteem of the young people by participation and encouraging them to use their ideas. The drama performance to their peers was a way of sharing the knowledge and experience that the young people had developed through the workshops.

The final drama production was faultless. The young people worked extremely hard in rehearsing and performing the drama piece. The performance lasted ten minutes and included two different scenes.

Staff were amazed at how well the young people progressed during the drama sessions. One young person at the beginning of the project refused to say anything – she would blush and run off. She was petrified of having to go on stage and it took a great deal of persuasion for her to be involved. Initially she had a very small part but by the end of the twenty weeks she was eager to take on a bigger role.

One of the young men worked really well on the drama throughout the length of the project. However, at the last minute he decided that he wasn't going to do the performance. He had felt very nervous and refused to go to the youth club to perform. It took one member of staff spending fifteen minutes talking through his concerns before he agreed to do it. After the performance he said it was nerve-racking but 'the best thing he had ever done'. The drama production was a tribute to the hard work of all the young people involved.

Using reflective practice

Many professionals and indeed health professionals are now encouraged to reflect on their practice. Staff in the project reflect 'on action'[9] i.e. is this working here and now – if not shall I change it? Similarly, we all reflected on action and all filled in a reflective log. This was a simple log of what we did, what went well and what we would do differently, if anything, next time. This informed evaluation and subsequent sessions. Finally, staff spent a short time at the end of each session reflecting on immediate thoughts and feelings and bringing back their reflections from the previous sessions.

Impact of the project

We believe that primary healthcare staff can successfully work with young people outside of a clinical setting. Not only has the project given the young people more information about their own health, but it has also taken them outside their own boundaries to experience life skills they otherwise would never have had the opportunity to experience. They may also feel more comfortable in accessing primary care services and, in particular, in discussing health issues with the practice nurse. As staff we have also stepped outside our own boundaries to share in that experience.

Continuing peer education

Many of the young people were keen to continue with the work and a Peer Education Programme took place over a residential weekend. Three girls and three boys took part at a youth hostel on the east coast. The residential was fully catered in order to give the young people the opportunity to focus on the work to be done. A full risk assessment was carried out prior to the weekend and appropriate insurance was obtained. The planned programme also included some leisure time.

Exercises aimed to provide them with the skills and experience to facilitate the '125 Health Project' workshop sessions to their peers at school. Having worked extremely hard over the residential weekend the young people produced their own resource pack to help them with the facilitation of the workshops. They planned what they would cover in the workshop sessions and who would say and do what. They used the resource pack and practised facilitating a workshop. The staff changed roles with the young people. The young people ran through the two different sessions using the staff to act as Year 7 pupils. This practice session was videoed. They then worked with staff to facilitate an introductory session and alcohol health workshop to their Year 7 peers.

Each individual learnt from the peer education training. Over the weekend the young people had increased in confidence and had enjoyed the training. The sessions that the young people facilitated were well received by their peers and many continued to support the programme after they had delivered their own sessions.

Mainstreaming of the work in education and health

The work has now developed across the city. The initial project team have formed a steering group to oversee the development of the work. Disseminating the project across key agencies has enabled the work to be mainstreamed. The 125 Health Project is now supported by the Sheffield Healthy School Standard. The local education authority's Access and Inclusion Department have encouraged the 'roll out' of the work and see the project as a model of good practice in working with vulnerable and challenging young people.

Following the development of a resource pack and training, the project has been 'rolled out' to several secondary schools across the city. This is included as part of the Health Improvement and Modernisation Programme and the Teenage Pregnancy Strategy and is supported by PCTs.

Integration in residential care

The project has also been delivered in a residential care home setting. The work was again evaluated and the new learning taken forward. As a result of this work the project is to be further piloted in three residential units. The main focus of the work in residential units will be building self-esteem and sexual health.

Conclusion

Never would the team have believed that a small pilot project could develop into something that is now becoming part of 'mainstream work' both in health and education in Sheffield. The key to success has been the determination of the team, creative engagement with young people, reflective practice and continuing evaluation demonstrating the impact that the project has had and is having on the lives of the young people involved.

References

1   Rosenfeld S (1996) Primary care experiences and preferences of urban youth. *J Paed Health Care.* **10**: 151–60.

2   Department of Health (1998) *Our Healthier Nation.* HMSO, London.

3   Department of Health (1998) *Smoking Kills.* HMSO, London.

4   Social Exclusion Unit (1999) *Reducing Teenage Pregnancy Report.* The Stationery Office, London.

5   Social Exclusion Unit (2001) *National Strategy for Neighbourhood Renewal. Report of Policy Action Team 12: Young People.* The Stationery Office, London.

6   Office of Population, Censuses and Surveys (1991) (Crown copyright) Central Policy Unit. Sheffield City Council.

7   Sheffield Hallam University (1995) *Safety On The Estates: A report on the conference.* Sheffield Hallam University, South Yorkshire Police, Sheffield City Council, Sheffield Housing and Sheffield Safer Cities.

8   Webster Stratton C (1994) *The Incredible Years, A Trouble Shooting Guide for Parents of Children aged 3–8 Years.* Umbrella Press, Onatrio.

9   Palmer A, Burns S and Bulman C (1994) *Reflective Practice in Nursing.* Blackwell Science, Oxford.

CHAPTER 10

Smoking cessation: a community education training programme

Bethan Plant and Juni Parkhurst

Introduction

Smoking is the single greatest cause of preventable illness and premature death in the UK.[1] It can occupy an important part of people's lives:

> 'Having a cigarette helps me get through the day. It calms me down, relaxes me and gives me five minutes peace and quiet away from the kids ... I know I should stop smoking and I understand that it's bad for my health but at the end of the day I don't do much for myself, I don't have much time to myself and I love catching up with my friends and having a cigarette. I don't spend money on other things for myself and I've tried to give up. It's dead hard, I can't do it – I suppose you'd say I'm addicted. Smoking is more than a habit for me it's also part of my life. I can get on with stuff if I know I've got a cigarette to look forward to.'

Adult smoking rates may be rising again.[1] Cigarette smoking appears to be a way of coping for people living in disadvantaged circumstances[2] where prevalence is disproportionately high.[1] Smoking has become a habit strongly associated with young, white, working-class women, particularly those on a low income with dependent children.[3] Stopping smoking, when it helps you 'get through', is not easy.[2] Smoking cessation support appropriate to needs is required but, apart from brief intervention advice, people are rarely given additional long-term help.

Primary care reality

Working in primary care and being expected to encourage and support people to stop smoking is challenging. Often people come in to see the practice nurse or doctor expecting him/her to wave a magic wand. Those who have tried to stop smoking and been unsuccessful, and those primary care staff who may have sought to help, often feel de-motivated and let down.

Primary care staff in disadvantaged communities are more aware than others that many people use smoking as a coping mechanism and they may feel uncomfortable about raising the issue of smoking. Offering appropriate advice and support requires sensitivity, persistence and innovative approaches.

The Community Education Training Programme

A Community Education Training Programme which has been run in Sheffield gives individuals the opportunity to attend smoking cessation support groups, which are facilitated by a primary care-based health professional and, crucially, a person living on an estate in a disadvantaged area who has been trained to provide smoking cessation support. The former is on hand to offer support and health advice and the latter 'community adviser' is available to encourage, motivate and counsel the group.

Advantage of community advisers

Involving and training local people to run smoking cessation groups empowers a member of the community in the transferable skills of group work and thus builds community resource. Having run one smoking cessation group and experienced the whole process, most people have felt ready to run more. Moreover, primary care professionals may be seen to lack understanding of the realities and difficulties of living on benefits and trying to stop smoking. In contrast a local person who has stopped smoking proves that it can be done.

Training community advisers

Anyone trained has to be a non-smoker, although often people have recently stopped smoking. Some are recruited through advertisements in the local GP practice or when attending smoking cessation groups run as part of the programme. The training takes a total of twenty hours. A payment of £25 is offered to individuals who train and each person is contracted to run at least two smoking cessation groups once they have completed the training.

'I saw a poster on the wall at the doctors. I'd recently stopped smoking myself. At first I didn't think I'd be any good at anything like this but I talked about it with a friend of mine who'd also just stopped. We both thought we'd give it a go. I know how hard it is to stop and I thought I might be able to help someone else. I have to admit being paid also encouraged me to find out more. It's not often we get opportunities like that round here.'

The aims of the training are to increase participants' confidence and self-esteem according to their learning styles, accessing the current skills of the participants and showing them how to exploit those skills. Participants should be left feeling they have the necessary skills, information and support to run a smoking cessation support group. Individuals are trained to run a group by providing them with a positive experience of a facilitated learning group, avoiding any hierarchical 'teacher/pupil' relationship, through three stages:

- dependency – on the group facilitator
- interdependency – on each other as sources of support
- independence – self-reliance and self-efficacy.

Process of training

Following introductions, a first exercise reveals everyone's historic relation-ship to smoking – whether people have smoked or not – and this usually relieves any fears among the participants. Often the group find that they have a lot in common and that their experiences are all valuable in helping to understand the difficulties associated with stopping smoking.

'I was really worried about the first training session. We were a fairly big group and I knew only one other person ... I was dreading having to speak up in front of everyone but it was really easy ... I was able to talk about what it was like when I stopped smoking and I can talk forever about that. I felt far more relaxed at the end.'

The training moves on to talk through the physiology and pharmacology of smoking. There is often a sense of shock – it is often the first time someone has explained exactly *why* and *how* smoking affects you. Participants are also introduced to the use of Nicotine Replacement Therapy, discussing the pros and cons of the different products that are available.

> 'I knew I had to stop smoking myself because I was always getting short of breath. But I couldn't believe all the other health problems that smoking can cause. I never knew there were 4000 different chemicals in cigarettes. I learnt loads when we did the session on health risks. I went home full of it, really fired up to help people to stop.'

Next, effective ways of helping people make behavioural changes are discussed, focusing upon individuals within the group who have had to make changes and looking at what helped or hindered. Positive affirmative language is used, e.g. 'stopping smoking' as opposed to 'giving up' which implies loss and sacrifice.

Training addresses participants' practice communication skills and their purpose in working with smokers (active listening, open and closed questions etc). Role play exercises are avoided except in circumstances where the role is set as participants often dislike and are uncomfortable with the 'acting' element. By now the group is usually well formed and individuals have developed a rapport. The group is able to hear different points of view, tolerate the way different personalities present themselves and communicate openly about problems and barriers to learning.

Theories of group life and dynamics are considered. Examples might be how to work with someone who talks too much, someone who is silent and someone who distracts and wants attention. Often individuals from local communities have very creative and effective ways of dealing with these situations, more so than health professionals who may be reluctant to take the initiative in dealing in a direct way with difficulties.

No work has to be carried out by participants in their own time as most are extremely busy and have no spare time during the course to do anything other than attend the training. The four-day course is usually timed so that it fits in with school hours, 10.30 am – 3.30 pm and so that the group can have lunch together. The social times are just as important as the formal teaching times.

Participants are moved gradually through exercises that require them to stand up and talk in front of other group members. This is often a new experience for many of the participants and the exercise helps improve confidence. In the penultimate session individuals are asked to prepare and facilitate a brief session – on a subject of their choice – followed by feedback on individual style and strengths. Some find this a major challenge but everyone gives each other support and the sense of achievement after the exercise is remarkable.

Implementing smoking cessation

In the final session the group look forward to what will happen after the course and what will be the first action that needs to be taken to establish the smoking cessation support groups. Each participant leaves with their own personalised plan of what they are going to do next.

Individuals are asked to set up a smoking cessation group in their local area. The local primary healthcare team is given details of the individuals who have trained in the area and groups are established which are run jointly and co-facilitated by the community adviser and a health visitor or practice nurse.

'At the end of the course I felt really pleased that I'd completed it. I felt dead proud of myself and I'd really enjoyed all the sessions. I was amazed how much I'd learnt and liked how we'd been taught. It wasn't like being in school or at college – I wasn't treated as though I was thick when I didn't understand stuff. I was a bit nervous about going on to run my smoking cessation group but in a way I was also looking forward to it.'

Tips and lessons from experience

Setting up a community adviser programme requires funding but initially a project can be targeted in one specific area and then developed according to resources available.

Recruiting group facilitators

The promotion of training through GP practices proved very successful. However, it is essential that people are clear about what the training involves and the commitment needed. Many would have a place booked on the training and then defaulted when they realised what was involved. To avoid this it is worth visiting individuals in their home to discuss the project. This gives people the opportunity to ask questions and to meet those involved. Avoid just sending letters, as literacy levels may be poor or people may be discouraged by long, detailed letters.

Training venues

Training venues have to be accessible bearing in mind that people may not be confident going to unfamiliar places or may need transport. It's often a good idea to choose a modern and comfortable venue. However, don't choose anywhere 'too posh' as it might make participants feel uncomfortable.

Payment to community advisers

This can be very difficult to organise. Individuals are often on low incomes or benefits and giving up a considerable amount of time to train as smoking cessation group facilitators. There must be an element of payment for those who complete the course but this needs to be considered so it does not affect benefit payments. Those attending the training in Sheffield received £25 at the end of the training and a further £25 when they had completed their first smoking cessation group.

Organising smoking cessation groups

Following the completion of the training there was difficulty in ensuring that individuals ran their own smoking cessation groups. As time elapsed people became less confident about facilitating the groups and some moved out of the area. It is important to organise local smoking cessation groups as soon as possible after the training has been completed.

After running the training in Sheffield, five community advisers who were trained went on to run their own smoking cessation groups. Originally, ten people started the initial training programme. Two people dropped out during the training and after the training ended one person moved out of the area and two people have gone on to take up full- or part-time employment.

What helped?

Training approach

The approaches and methods used take account of participants feeling uncomfortable and anxious about working in groups and the training encourages individuals' confidence to grow throughout the course.

Support from primary healthcare staff

Those individuals who were most successful in the training and with running smoking cessation groups were those who received valuable support from a member of their local primary care team. Some individuals had been encouraged to train as facilitators by their practice nurse or health visitor and some had also pre-arranged to run groups locally with the practice nurse or health visitor when they had completed the training. This worked really well.

Linking with others

Specialist smoking cessation support services now operate across the country. Any community adviser programme needs to integrate with local specialist cessation support services. The focus in Sheffield is to continue to run the community advisers programme and to recruit new advisers. In the future it is hoped that the model of training community advisers can be expanded and operated across the whole city.

The training programme requires a great deal of organisation and involves many different agencies. In particular, it develops a strong link between primary care and the local community. Moreover, the project encourages joint working between primary care trusts, city-wide Specialist Smoking Cessation Support Service and local GP practices.

What impact has the project had?

The project has made a positive impact in a number of ways. Links between primary care and the local community have been developed further. Health professionals involved have developed good links with individuals living in the area through their role in co-facilitating groups, while local residents have felt more comfortable in approaching primary care staff.

In particular, the training has enhanced local skills and increased confidence and self-esteem. Most individuals finish the training and many go on to co-facilitate a number of different groups. Some have gone on to enrol on other courses run by the local colleges. Last, but not least, the Community Adviser Programme has been very successful in supporting individuals who want to stop smoking.

Evaluation of the work

Evaluation using focus groups with individuals who have attended smoking cessation groups has indicated that the approach used and the combination of a health professional and local person jointly facilitating the groups works extremely well and is much valued. Group members have stated that the community adviser has provided on-going support by visiting people or having a chat with group members when he/she has seen them out shopping. It is clear that the community advisers have also played an extremely important role in recruiting local people to the groups and also motivating individuals.

> 'When I joined the group, I didn't know anybody. I'd never met anybody or seen anybody in this group before except the community adviser. She's been really good because she's been policing us while we've been out of the group. If she's seen me out and about on the estate she's always asked how I'm doing and how I am feeling. I think she's good because it is this area where we come from and she relates directly to us. The community adviser and practice nurse complement each other because they both support and help us.'

Conclusion: further messages

Initially, establish the project on a small scale and develop the work as a pilot project, targeting a number of disadvantaged areas and tailoring training to meet the needs of the individuals who are attending. In particular, ensure that a trainer is recruited who has experience in working with and training people from local communities. The trainer has to be able to communicate with people on all levels and the bottom line is that the trainer makes the project a success. The participants need to feel comfortable with the trainer.

- **Don't expect too much too soon.** For many people attending the training this is a whole new experience. Individuals' confidence will grow but don't push people too far too soon. People will feel more comfortable running groups when they have more experience – don't encourage people to run two or three groups at a time straight away.
- **Offer continuing support to community advisers.** Once individuals have completed the training, arrange to meet up regularly so that the training group continues to meet together for peer support and to talk through their experiences of running their own smoking cessation groups.

- **Be sure to evaluate**. Ensure that the project is based on research and evidence based practice. Carry out focus groups with the community advisers, health professionals and those individuals who have attended the smoking cessation groups. And then act on recommendations!

References

1   Department of Health (1998) *'Smoking Kills': A White Paper on Tobacco*. The Stationery Office, London.

2   Blackburn C and Graham H (1992) *Smoking Among Working Class Mothers. Information Pack*. Department of Applied Social Studies, University of Warwick, Coventry.

3   Graham H (1989) Women and Smoking in the United Kingdom: The Implications for health promotion. *Health Promotion Journal* 3(4): 317–82.

CHAPTER 11

Second Chancers: community cardiac rehabilitation in the inner city

Ann Potter

Responding to local need

The disadvantaged inner west of Newcastle upon Tyne gained national notoriety during the riots of 1991 in Benwell. It has high levels of unemployment, with the majority of people living in rented housing.[1] Most of the city's South Asian households reside in west Newcastle with a 25–30% increased incidence of ischaemic heart disease (IHD).[2] In 1996 mortality and morbidity of IHD in west Newcastle was the highest in the district with age standardised death rates for males under 75 at 235, with a district figure of 201. Yet coronary revascularisation rates were the lowest across the district at 6.6 per 10 000 compared to 10.2 per 10 000 elsewhere in the district.[3] Moreover, take up of existing rehabilitation services by local people appeared poor.

A pioneering healthy living centre, the West End Health Resource Centre in Benwell, targets such high risk and vulnerable groups. Opened by Tony Blair in 1996, the centre, a charitable trust, provides a well-equipped gym and studio, traditional therapies, e.g. physiotherapy, and the provision of alternative therapies such as reflexology and aromatherapy. Aiming to deliver health messages in a more positive and meaningful way, the centre is testing the benefits of new approaches to health needs. Innovations have included an anxiety and exercise programme and sessions for a head injury support group.

Piloting community cardiac rehabilitation

A pilot, funded by the health authority, began in June 1997. Working closely with the local acute hospital unit, post myocardial infarction (MI) patients were identified on admission and offered locally based cardiac rehabilitation. Over a nine-month period 76 people were referred. Initially, the targeted area covered a locality of 13 general practices serving 84 000 people.

Following home-based assessment and support, the patient and partner/friend attended a ten-week group programme at West End Health Resource Centre. Information from follow-up assessments at six months was fed back to their primary care teams to support chronic disease management. A high degree of co-morbidity was identified (28% claiming incapacity benefit) with a number of 'hard to reach' individuals requiring additional flexible support, for example a man living in a bail hostel. The pilot demonstrated a need for sensitive, locally based services in the community with a high up-take of these services when provided – 75% attended the group programme.

With the formation of Newcastle West PCG the area covered by the programme grew to encompass 16 GP practices with 114 000 practice population. Newcastle West PCG funded the project from 1998 to 2001 following the initial pilot.

Why do cardiac rehabilitation?

Cardiac rehabilitation reduces mortality and morbidity, improves quality of life and enhances secondary prevention of coronary heart disease (CHD).[4] A meta-analysis of 22 randomised trials demonstrated a 20–25% reduction in mortality.[5,6] A reduction of 50% in anxiety and depression scores was demonstrated following introduction of the *Heart Manual*.[7]

Unfortunately in the UK there has been poor provision and take up of cardiac rehabilitation services which often targeted low-risk white male post MI patients.[8] Attendance at rehabilitation programmes remains low, involving only 25% of all experiencing MI and 10% of angioplasty patients.[9] The recent national service framework (NSF) for IHD has set milestones for national provision – 85% of patients, post MI, to be offered rehabilitation.[10]

Aim of rehabilitation

The aim of cardiac rehabilitation is to facilitate physical, psychological and emotional recovery, improve functional capacity and enable patients to achieve and maintain better health. Rehabilitation is usually described in phases. Phase 1 (4–5 days) begins in hospital following medical management and stabilisation and is when patients are given an explanation and understanding of their disease.

Once discharged, a gradual exercise programme begins in Phase II (4–6 weeks) with psychological assessment and support to elicit health beliefs and cardiac misconceptions, helping to re-frame these beliefs. The *Heart Manual* approach follows a cognitive behavioural model and provides a relaxation and stress management programme for post MI patients. Throughout the process vocational/social issues are addressed. Phase II is usually home based and involves other family members.

The emphasis in Phase III (6–16 weeks post MI) is on a supervised group-based course, held at the Resource Centre or an alternative leisure facility. A structured and individual exercise programme is delivered, informal discussions are held and there is support from specialists, e.g. dieticians, covering a wide variety of health information.

Phase IV is about the long term, hopefully maintaining the gains and life-style changes achieved, supported by family/friends and primary care. 'Cardiac rehab puts you on the right track – it's up to you to keep it going and not go off the rails.'

Improving access with a community model

Traditional rehabilitation programmes offer an outpatient group where patients are invited to return to the hospital, commencing about six weeks after the event. Yet feelings of uncertainty and vulnerability are most acute in the immediate post-discharge period and intervention at this time is highly valued by patients and their families. Patients often feel more relaxed and familiar with a community facility. There may also be difficulties in accessing a hospital service due to the geographical location, the language/cultural needs of some patients and for those with physical/sensory disability.

Adopting a flexible approach

The rehabilitation process encourages active participation in healthcare in contrast to becoming a passive recipient. Many disadvantaged individuals find it hard to 'grasp the nettle' having limited feelings of control over the situation. Previous life experiences, co-morbidity of mental or physical ill health and social/cultural issues have significant impact on the individual's health beliefs, life choices and feelings of self control. Some have adapted to the constraints of chronic illness rather than learnt therapeutic measures of self care.

In order to make an impact on health outcomes the service has to be sensitive to these issues, providing flexibility based on individual need, instead of a service led programme. This approach is time consuming, but is essential if it is to make a real difference. For example, negotiating very small but achievable goals with some clients to increase confidence and functional ability; supporting those who are uncomfortable in a group situation by the provision of fringe activities; acknowledging that some individuals, although well aware of the health risks of smoking, are still at the contemplative stage, requiring appropriate support and encouragement or accepting that the time between rehabilitation phases may differ and should be needs led.

Programme Development

A series of planning meetings with representatives from hospital and community in collaboration with other agencies led to the initiation of this community rehabilitation programme. The project has been steered by a multi-disciplinary group with representatives from a users group (heart support group) and the Resource Centre. Initially focusing on post MI patients, there was a gradual introduction of those who had had revascularisation, particularly coronary artery by-pass grafts. Some angina patients who needed support to make lifestyle changes were also accepted.

People involved

During this period (1998–2001) the core rehabilitation team, engaged in all phases of the rehabilitation process, consisted of two experienced community nurses and a part-time administrator. The programme was supported by a community cardiologist, the multi-disciplinary steering group and the management team at the West End Health Resource Centre. The Phase III exercise programme was provided by the exercise team, physiotherapy in conjunction with the nursing team, and health topics were covered by dieticians, pharmacists, cardiologists, physiotherapists, psychologists and Second Chancers (heart support group).

Figure 11.1 shows the increase in referrals between 1998 and 2000.

Pathway of care

Community cardiac rehabilitation provides continuity during Phase II through to Phase IV with feedback to GP practices at six weeks and six

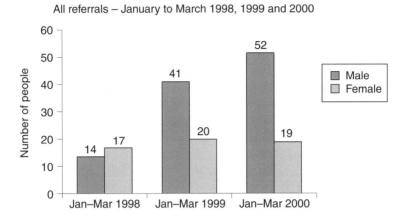

All referrals – January to March 1998, 1999 and 2000

Figure 11.1 Cardiac rehabilitation programme – referrals.

months and has close communication links with the acute units. Patients are introduced to the programme by the nursing team whilst in hospital.

Individual home-based assessment and support are offered to all patients and their families. Where appropriate, the *Heart Manual* programme is the structured tool offered to post MI patients with adapted and translated material for South Asian clients. Assessments of physical and emotional recovery, identification of co-morbidity, support with lifestyle changes, e.g. smoking cessation, and a programme of increasing physical activity form part of the Phase II intervention. During this period the group based Phase III programme is introduced with a future appointment negotiated.

Phase III – the rehabilitation group

Community rehabilitation offers an eight or ten week rolling programme of group rehabilitation. Sessions are held either in the Resource Centre or at a local leisure centre. Each two-hour session includes an individual exercise programme, relaxation session and covers a series of health topics. Examples include 'stress management', 'cholesterol and fats', 'what is heart disease?' and 'moving on'. Whilst initially receiving intensive support to complete the exercise circuit, independence is encouraged. Before the group sessions are completed the rehabilitation team encourage participants to join general resource centre exercise and fitness sessions.

An interview at the end of the course considers lifestyle changes made and negotiates realistic maintenance of those changes with the client. At the rehab group in 1998–1999, 60% were high attenders at 6–10 sessions, 21% low attenders at 1–5 sessions, and 12% failed to attend. A review at six months assesses symptoms and functional status, lifestyle and coronary risk factors, medication compliance and side effects. Psychological status is determined using the hospital anxiety and depression score and a question about quality of life. This information is collated and also fed back to the patient's GP.

Case example: Bob's experiences of community cardiac rehabilitation

Bob was introduced to the programme by a member of the team whilst he was still in hospital. He was recovering from his fourth MI. At 58-years-old he had angina and left ventricular failure, reasonably controlled with medication although his functional ability was significantly impaired. Despite striving to make lifestyle changes following previous MIs, Bob admitted that he remained a 'smoking couch potato'. With no previous rehabilitation he received intensive support once discharged with weekly home visits to provide smoking cessation counselling, to facilitate the *Heart Manual* and to encourage a gradual exercise programme. His carbon monoxide levels were measured at each visit and he realised the immediate effect of his smoking cessation which he later attributed as one of the reasons for his success. At six weeks post MI he entered the group programme and found the peer support invaluable. As he had poor left ventricular function and angina on moderate exertion, his exercise programme was tailored accordingly. Bob enjoyed the support and activities of the group and made close friends with two other group members, eventually becoming founder members of Second Chancers. Initially, Bob was informed by the medical team that he was to be referred for heart transplant, but on subsequent assessment he was 'too fit to necessitate a transplant' and has since undergone coronary artery by-pass grafts. Two years after referral to the programme Bob remains an ex-smoker, exercises regularly at the Resource Centre and is an active member of Second Chancers. He firmly believes that his previous lifestyle had a significant impact on the outcome of his disease and with appropriate support at an earlier stage the deterioration in his cardiac function would have been prevented.

Smoking cessation

Individual smoking cessation support is available to all in the programme. Using the Prochaska and DiClementi Change Cycle motivation and readiness to change are assessed with appropriate interventions. The use of a carbon monoxide smokerlyser reinforces the health benefits to those who have recently stopped smoking.

For those who remain highly motivated but are struggling, specialist support is offered. Patients are offered counselling following a behavioural approach and assessed for NRT. More recently, we have been able to refer to the smoking clinics developed in GP practices. Figure 11.2 shows reduction in smoking for MI patients.

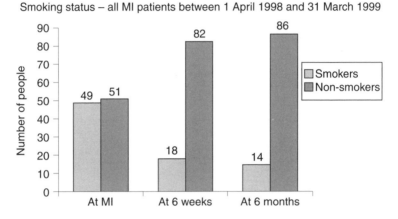

Figure 11.2   Cardiac rehabilitation programme – smoking status.

Challenges for the work

Most Phase III cardiac rehab programmes are held in the acute setting with guidelines from the British Association of Cardiac Rehabilitation recommending a venue with medical and emergency back up. We needed to assure the safety and effectiveness of our approach in the community.

Developing and sustaining effective communication

Good communication links with all primary healthcare teams were essential to raise awareness of our work and find the best method of sharing information. Initially, we conducted practice visits, backed up with written material and newsletters. However, it was patient feedback that made the most impact.

Communication with key personnel in secondary care had begun when planning the pilot. This was continued with regular visits to the local coronary care unit (CCU) and 'step-down' ward. The recent appointment of a rehabilitation co-ordinator in the cardio-thoracic unit should ensure comprehensive coverage for patients. In addition there have been joint training programmes for primary and secondary care staff involved. The latter are also represented on the district cardiac rehabilitation group, and involved in local strategic development of rehabilitation services and implementation of the NSF.

Improving equity

Psychosocial factors can have a significant impact on outcomes of cardiac disease. In 1998–1999 51% of our referrals, for people who were pre-retirement, were either unemployed or on incapacity benefit. We are conscious that nationally there remains less rehabilitation provision for women, older people, disadvantaged groups and minority ethnic groups.

It will take time and realistic resource to provide an equitable service for disadvantaged groups. Provision must be needs led with a flexible approach. For example, someone with learning disabilities may need more individual support over an extended period with provision to increase time spent in the group.

Case examples

Harry was agoraphobic, he panicked at the thought of social contact. It took weeks to get him into the centre and a further period to get him onto the fringe of the group. Gradually he has joined the group when exercising and now joins in the health discussions.

Joan was post MI with diabetes, hypertension, obesity and arthritis. Although physical activity can produce a feeling of well being and an increase in functional ability and stamina, this process takes time. The potential impact on Joan's existing conditions was discussed and the exercise programme was extended until Joan became aware of the benefits with a noticeable improvement in mobility and stamina.

People from South Asian communities

Vigorous attempts were made to address the language and cultural barriers of South Asian patients. It has been necessary to tailor the service to indivi-

dual needs, e.g. interpreters are requested with allocation of longer appointment times; the need to provide transport to the sessions for fear of racism –
intimidation is met with the provision of taxis. These additional costs have
been funded separately through a charitable funding source.

Close collaboration with another local project employing bi-lingual health
development workers led to joint assessment visits with a rehabilitation
team member. Where appropriate the health development worker accompanied the patient to the initial exercise sessions, when future interpreting and
support needs were assessed. A resource file of written, audio and video
material translated into the main South Asian languages reinforced the
health and information messages.

Despite these measures we are not yet adequately meeting the needs of
this group. A recent *New Deal for Communities* bid was successful and will
support a project designed to identify the needs of the South Asian community with existing or at risk of IHD that has just been launched and can link
with the existing rehabilitation system.

Working in the voluntary sector

The Resource Centre is a voluntary sector project that had management and
budgetary responsibility for the rehabilitation programme. The culture and
previous experience of staff from statutory agencies can differ from those in
the voluntary sector with the potential for conflict. Thus, it seemed essential
that those planning the exercise component should be health personnel
with some previous experience of outpatient cardiac rehabilitation. The
physiotherapist and rehabilitation co-ordinator planned the sessions,
neglecting to include experienced exercise specialists who were part of the
Resource Centre team and who initially didn't feel any ownership of the
programme. Open debate has resolved the tensions.

Similarly, setting up a specialist smoking service for rehabilitation patients
created concern for voluntary sector management. They worried that the
local community and centre users would interpret this as a victim-blaming
or anti-smoking strategy. Once it became apparent that the clinic was
meeting an expressed need of our client group these concerns diminished.

What helped?

Planning and joint working

Six months of discussion and planning with multi-disciplinary representatives from a range of agencies preceded the introduction of the programme

and led to a project steering group. The sharing of knowledge and expertise in support of this programme made a real difference. So often there is professional jealousy and protectiveness, which creates barriers to the successful development of new initiatives.

Sharing skills

This type of work requires specific skills and experiences. Some knowledge of cardiology and experience in a CCU is helpful although not essential. Nevertheless, it is important to update on the modern management of IHD. A knowledge and experience of the community, available resources and an understanding of community development are a distinct advantage. Skills in motivational interviewing, smoking cessation counselling and group work are also required. These are skills that many nurses with a community background may possess.

User feedback

Patients are the best advocates, feeding back their experiences and outcomes of the rehabilitation process to GPs and cardiologists. Once the project's value is understood and accepted and confidence raised, so referrals increase. Gradually the local community became aware of the programme and, as word spread, self-referrals began.

Job satisfaction

Although challenging, demanding and at times stressful work, job satisfaction eases the burden. It is very satisfying to see the impact this approach has on patient outcomes and quality of life.

Impact of the programme

For families and community

> 'If I'd been offered rehabilitation years ago I'm sure I would not have had further heart attacks.'

Patients who had not been offered rehabilitation support following previous acute cardiac events have reported that, had rehabilitation been available, their outcomes would have been very different. Many believe that with appropriate interventions following a previous MI they would not have suffered further attacks or required revascularisation procedures.

The diagnosis of MI can have a profound effect on the patient and family, causing fears that any future employment is in jeopardy or that their life will never be the same again. Resuming employment, regaining confidence and fitness and reducing risk factors are common rehabilitation outcomes. Some have the motivation and support to achieve these goals by their own endeavours but others require support and encouragement through this difficult time.

Case example

Eddie and Violet felt they had missed out on the previous three years following Eddie's serious MI. They lived in fear, unable to engage in past activities. This couple then attended the rehabilitation group together and gradually their confidence increased. They now feel back to normal and describe rehabilitation as a 'miracle'.

'Second Chancers' – the self-help group

Within the first year past and present patients set up a self-help and social group. 'Second Chancers' is now an independent group organising social events, walks and fund raising activities. Members have offered individual support to those recently diagnosed when requested and had an active voice on the programme steering group and the Resource Centre managing group.

Second Chancers have fund raised to provide an automatic defibrillator for the rehab centres. Cardio-pulmonary resuscitation training, already offered to patients and relatives, has also been provided for local shopkeepers and businesses.

Disseminating health messages locally

Working locally and with other family members helps to disseminate health messages into the local community. By utilising and building on existing local services we can help to create sustainable change. In the future it is hoped that the skills and expertise of Second Chancers, as people who are affected by this chronic disease, can be developed to support others.

Impact for providers and service development

For primary and secondary care the need for a flexible cardiac rehabilitation service has been highlighted. It is now recognised that a locally based programme is safe and effective, with increased uptake and improved outcomes especially for disadvantaged communities.

In 2001 the success of this programme led to the expansion of the service across the whole of Newcastle upon Tyne co-ordinated by a newly appointed nurse consultant in cardiac rehabilitation who replaced the existing nurse specialist on her retirement. In the longer term it is anticipated that the majority of patients with a range of cardiac conditions will be offered cardiac rehabilitation in their local community while they are high-risk patients.

Conclusion

This initiative is now an integral part of the effective care and prevention of heart disease in Newcastle. It has been essential to have everyone on board during the planning stages. The programme encourages individuals to take control and become active participants, not passive recipients. It provides continuity over an extended period of time for users, bridging the gap between primary and secondary care. For success the service has had to be needs led and offer flexibility to address the complex and varying needs of disadvantaged communities.

References

1   Newcastle City Council (1997) *City Profiles. Results from the 1996 inter-censal survey*. Chief Executive's Department, NCC, Newcastle.

2   The Newcastle Strategy Group (1996) *Taking Heart*. University of Newcastle-upon-Tyne.

3   Directorate of Public Health (1997) *Health Profiles by Locality*. Newcastle and North Tyneside Health Authority.

4   Thompson DR, Bowman GS, *et al*. (1996) Cardiac rehabilitation in the United Kingdom: guidelines and audit standards. *Heart*. **75**: 89–93.

5   O'Connor GT, Burning JE, Yusuf S, *et al*. (1998) An overview of randomised trials of rehabilitation with exercise after myocardial infarction. *Circulation*. **80**: 234–44.

6   Oldridge NB, Guyatt GH, *et al*. (1988) Cardiac rehabilitation after myocardial infarction: combined experience of randomised controlled trials. *JAMA*. **260**: 945–50.

7   Lewin B, Robertson IH, *et al.* (1992) Effects of self-help post myocardial infarction, rehabilitation on psychological adjustment and the use of health services. *Lancet.* **339**: 1036–40.

8   Thompson DR, Bowman GS, Kitson AL, *et al.* (1997) Cardiac rehabilitation services in England and Wales: a national survey. *Cardiology.* **59**: 229–304.

9   Bethell HJN, Taylor SC, *et al.* (2001) Cardiac rehabilitation in the United Kingdom. How complete is the provision? *J Cardiopulm Rehabil.* **21**: 111–15.

10   Department of Health (2000) National Service Framework for Coronary Heart Disease. DOH, London.

CHAPTER 12

A whole system approach to change in mental health services: throwing stones or throwing birds?

Dave Tomson and Steve Nash

Introduction

This chapter is a 'warts and all' story about work to encourage a shift towards an integrated primary care and community model for delivery of mental health services in a part of northeast England. We hope that it will be interesting and useful to others addressing change.

National context

Mental health services currently have a high policy priority with new plans and guidance afoot.[1] Key themes are shown in Box 12.1.

Apparent failures in management of people with long-term mental illness promote a safety and risk reduction agenda for government. Meanwhile, primary care is criticised for poor identification and management of people with mental distress. Service users express widespread dissatisfaction with services and ways of working.[2] Morale amongst mental health service providers in both specialist and generalist settings is low, with staff recruitment and retention dwindling.[3]

Box 12.1: Policy themes for mental health services

- New National Standards, including a new emphasis on the importance of primary care.[4]
- New performance management and accountability frameworks.[5]
- Emphasis on partnerships, particularly with social services and the voluntary sector.
- Emphasis on workforce planning linking training to service needs.[6]
- Renewed emphasis on flexible working patterns and multidisciplinary training.[6]
- Increasing involvement of users, carers and public in planning, delivery and monitoring.
- Healthy Living Centres[7] and new importance attached to mental health promotion.
- Policy implementation guides – blueprints for local service configuration.

Epidemiology of mental ill health

The prevalence of identified and diagnosed mental health problems is increasing, and is much greater in disadvantaged settings.[8] An adult has a one in three lifetime risk of having diagnosable mental illness, and mental health difficulties are the predominant issue in over 30% of all consultations in primary care. Up to 50% of all persons with a severe and disabling mental illness were seen exclusively in inner city primary care rather than specialist mental health services[8] with over 90% seeing their GP in the previous year.[9]

'Family support workers are constantly dealing with people who have attempted suicide over the weekend. I am alarmed at the number of people I see with mental health problems. None of them go to the community mental health team. Some don't have a GP. We don't need the medical model in the community – we need an army of barefoot community workers.'

Health Visitor

Mental health and social disadvantage

Material and social deprivation, financial hardship, and widening discrepancies in relative wealth are associated with, and probably contribute to, a greater prevalence of mental ill health in the inner city.[8] Poverty and unemployment increase the duration of common mental disorders, and are also associated with a higher prevalence of psychosis and admission to psychiatric hospital.[8-10] Financial strain appears a predictor of future mental ill health[11] as does a low standard of living.[12-14] Poverty or severe economic loss is associated with higher rates of mental illness and antisocial behaviour in children, although cultural factors may protect some ethnic groups.

> 'People on the borderlines do not fit – those with personality problems, or drug and alcohol problems or learning difficulties in addition to mental illness – teams and wards won't work with them. The voluntary sector ends up taking responsibility for those who do not fit neat categories.'
>
> *Community Support Worker*

Need for change

For those patients in two neighbouring primary care localities on Tyneside (previously primary care groups of Riverside in North Tyneside and East in Newcastle) access to specialist mental health services had been based wholly on diagnostic categories, as often occurs elsewhere. Thus, only those labelled with severe psychiatric illness were seen. In addition, there was no access to crisis intervention. This created tensions between primary and secondary care.

Many, including service users, community workers and primary care professionals, felt the configuration and culture of local mental health services needed review. The new emphasis on a 'primary care led NHS' and emerging interest in whole system methods offered the promise of tackling the problem.

Whole system approach

A definition of a system is an organisation forming a network especially for distributing something or serving a common purpose. A whole system intervention typically involves representative stakeholders meeting to discuss work that was previously reserved for 'those at the top'.

Whole systems interventions assume that everyone, rather than just experts, is required for whole system change. In whole systems work, a set of people, needs and services are seen as an interconnected whole. There is an emphasis on collaboration and partnership, on living relationships and networks, on finding creative ways to explore possibilities and on agreeing sustainable ways of tackling problems that may otherwise overwhelm individual agencies.

What we set out to do

Locally there was considerable momentum for an approach that considered the local mental health system as an organic whole – so that social, community and needs-based perspectives could be considered alongside psychiatric and medical models. Such an approach would challenge the dominant mythology that specialist services saw all the serious illness, whilst primary care saw only the 'worried well'. There was also a conviction that the existing system did not maximise the capacity and expertise available, especially in primary care. Most of all, the system did not make sense from a service user perspective. We kept in mind a set of principles that we thought it was important to incorporate (*see* Box 12.2).

Box 12.2: Core principles used

- People want services in non-stigmatising primary and community settings where possible.[15]
- Solutions should be whole system and owned by users, workers and planners.
- Solutions should be 'both' rather than either/or.
- Much more sharing of language, culture, aims and objectives is needed.
- Partnership means mutuality with all partners sharing responsibility for the whole problem.
- Concentrate on process and function not structure.
- Move from the language of 'primary and secondary care' to 'generalists and specialists'.
- Community development and wider networks (self help and community resources) are crucial to the results.
- Aim for increased capacity in both formal and informal care systems.
- Move from ideas of outreach to inreach – the use of the hospital is just one of a range of interventions.
- Referral means 'yours not mine', consultation means 'let's think and work together'.
- Model of care should incorporate the best of medical, psychological and social models.
- Listen to service users and carers – cross check all developments against this principle.

A three-phase plan

A Whole System Mental Health Project was envisaged in three phases. The first phase included an extensive mapping exercise, followed by a whole system event (see below). Phase two was expected to focus on service reconfiguration (informed by the whole system event) and would feature a great deal of change management, education, training and capacity building in primary care mental health work. Finally, in phase three it was expected that a whole system approach to service commissioning would be in place and that the lessons learned would be translated into deliverable programmes for utilisation elsewhere.

What happened?

Service mapping for elephant problems

This included over 80 interviews with individuals and groups from primary care, community mental health teams, services users and voluntary and community agencies. The quotes throughout this chapter are from this mapping exercise. Participants were asked: 'When you think about the system of mental health services locally, what concerns you most?' Results were grouped to define a set of 'elephant problems'.

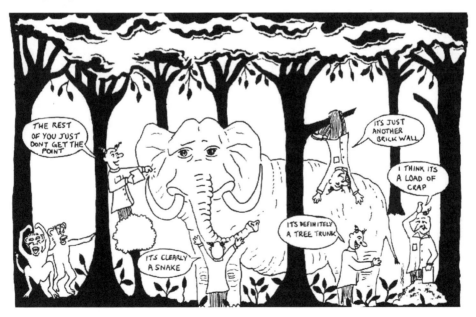

'"Elephant problems" are so called because of their size, messiness and their tendency to appear to be different depending on your perspective. It follows that progress is only likely once a shared (whole system) view is arrived at. In the above illustration different professionals and providers struggle to agree what the problems are and what needs to be done to solve them.'

Illustration by Rob Belilios, mental health service user

Elephant problems identified included:

- lack of a clear, comprehensive and integrated vision for local services – so new resources are simply 'bolted on' to a fragmented system
- no common language or culture – no agreed consensus about priorities
- conflict over disability v diagnosis-based ways of working[8]; no sense of common ownership over care protocols and pathways
- quality of care is unpredictable and inconsistent, especially where similar services are managed by different providers e.g. counselling and clinical psychology in primary care; long waiting times
- interface issues between primary care and specialist mental health, especially around threshold of access and 'border disputes' about responsibilities for differing needs[8]
- repeat assessments for service users, who ended up feeling 'bounced around' the system[15]
- variable levels of mental health expertise, resource and capacity across different general practices
- lack of information about what is available and how to access it.

'When the police are involved, they always come mob handed. They used handcuffs on me in front of my 12-year-old son. I was sitting there calmly – my son tried to hit the officer and is now set against them. Ward 21 sent me home half an hour later.'

Service user

Whole system event

In May 2000 a whole system event (WSE) involved 150 people meeting together to focus on problems and successes of the existing system and to define the changes and actions required. Some of the common themes that emerged were a pressing need for:

- equity of access to services at all levels
- a common language for priorities and needs

- agreed protocols and pathways between services
- integrated community and primary care resources
- shared multi-disciplinary/multi-agency training
- access to choice and non-medical alternatives
- recognition of service user and carer expertise
- a whole system approach.

What happened next?

We had enabled the development of a 'bottom up' and primary care led agenda for the reconfiguration of local mental health services. However, we had underestimated how threatening this would be to the statutory and specialist part of the system.

We engaged with a wide selection of stakeholders, but we did not get sufficient ownership at board level in the mental health trust – those with most power were least involved. Enthusiasm for change was seen as uninformed radicalism. As a result, the consultation exercise and WSE were not discussed by those with influence over the future development of services.

At the same time, a far less predictable problem occurred. The project's sole worker became seriously ill and there was no-one with the necessary time and energy to follow up on the specific actions of the WSE.

Phases two and three

Despite attempts to maintain the energy and momentum of the project, colleagues at all levels became preoccupied by other changes that at times threatened to overwhelm. These included the standards and performance targets of the National Service Framework for Mental Health published at the end of 1999, creation of a new specialist mental health trust, and the two primary care groups heading towards two separate primary care trusts.

We could not stick to the original plan but the creation of a new mental health trust brought some new faces and fresh thinking. The importance of developing a whole system approach, and the related acceptance of the needs and contribution of primary care were openly acknowledged and to a certain extent promoted at a senior level. The shift towards a primary care trust also offered new possibilities, not least because some of the resources providing therapeutic input in general practice (e.g. counselling and clinical psychology) were now employed by the new PCT.

Plan B

The programme was revised to include the following.

- Set up and support a primary care mental health facilitator role, to undertake audit and education initiatives at the level of individual practices starting to implement the NSF for Mental Health.
- Focus on the interface between primary care, community development and mental health, including hosting a regional conference, developing a primary care mental health user group and using a brief therapy approach to piloting a stress and exercise group in a community gym.
- Project management of a service development bid for a new model of psychological therapies in primary care.

Of these, the development of a psychological therapies model was most in keeping with the original objective to enable the reconfiguration of resources. The next section considers this initiative and its outcomes.

> 'GPs don't know enough. I've been on antidepressants for five years, since I was 15. I wanted help with panic attacks and was told I could see a psychologist in six months, so got more tablets. I always end up nearly in tears when I leave the surgery.'
>
> *Service user*

A Primary Care Psychological Therapies Model

We were keen to create a new role for multi-skilled workers (specialist mental health workers) who would be core to primary care teams. They would provide as many of the following functions for effective primary mental health care as possible.

- Effective triage and timely initial assessment.
- A broad range of psychosocial interventions – evidence based.
- Information giving, self-help materials, signposting, community networks.
- Education and training for primary care teams to increase skill and capacity.
- Supervision, consultation and support for primary care teams.
- Research, audit and databases regarding mental health work.
- Clear protocols and pathways with specialist and other services.

What actually happened?

We underestimated the degree of political sensitivity involved in the proposals. Commissioning was being transferred from the local health authority to the new PCT and we were perceived to be acting exclusively for primary care. There were major concerns that psychological therapies in primary care would be prioritised above other important needs, and before new structures were in place. Furthermore, it proved difficult to get consensus on the notion of a core worker with a broad range of skills.

Despite these barriers, a great deal of awareness raising and debate had occurred with greater currency for whole systems principles. Primary care teams had to think long and hard about the kind of resources and service models they wanted. New investment was eventually won for primary care mental health work, and in fact this development received the lion's share of the available investment monies for 2002–2003. The management and support of the proposed new workers were taken on by the specialist mental health trust, given that the very new PCT did not have the capacity.

External evaluation of project impact

Preliminary findings indicated the failure to get sufficient ownership by all the major stakeholders at the beginning and this compromised the project's ability to achieve its goals. Other limiting factors included the lack of specific action planning and follow up to the WSE, and the decision to take on a project management role for psychological therapies with the apparent loss of political neutrality.

The main achievements relate to the way in which the project team brought 'vision and passion to mental health services'. The project has acted as a catalyst for change, through the way it has challenged traditionally held values and assumptions about mental health services. It has raised the profile of mental health beyond the traditional boundaries of specialist mental health services.

Moreover, existing tensions are out in the open and this has helped create an environment for change in working across organisational boundaries. People are more likely to avoid simple couplings such as 'severe mental illness is for specialists' and 'common mental health problems are for generalists'. Instead, people are more likely to talk of consultation and not just referral.

We may have 'softened people to embrace new concepts' (from an evaluation interview). We introduced new values by focusing on needs rather than diagnosis. We highlighted that there were in effect two separate mental health systems operating, in primary and secondary care. These challenges to existing orthodoxy are seen as facilitating more recent initiatives introduced by the Specialist Mental Health Trust.

Other successes include engaging service user groups and voluntary sector organisations. Our introduction of specialist mental health workers in primary care is seen as having a positive impact and having been well received by primary care practitioners.

Lessons for the future

Starting out

- Be as clear as possible about the intention. If it's about entering into a whole system process with genuine curiosity and trust in the approach then the project needs to be as neutral as possible. If it's really about developing services in one part of the system then be honest about this at the outset.
- Ensure that all the key players are signed up at the appropriate hierarchical levels.
- Establish at the outset what is to be done with any reports or recommendations, i.e. where they are to be presented.
- Be realistic about the scope of the work – better to cover one geographical locality well than to struggle to cover two.
- Whole systems working is time and energy consuming. Do not underestimate the demands that this will make on the local system – lack of commitment, or preoccupation with structural changes will diminish the capacity that people will have to engage with the process.

Facilitating the process

- Get a really good map of the local system – services, gaps and relationships, perceptions, communication lines, pathways, effective partnerships, border disputes, decision-making processes, committee structure.
- Try also to focus on what works well – what do people want to keep?
- Take time to establish dialogue, especially where polarised views exist. It's possible to jump to holding a WSE before the different parties are ready to engage as partners.
- Consider offering training, e.g. for service users, to act as facilitators for the process or at stakeholder events.
- Consider a series of stakeholder conferences instead of a one-off event.

• Be aware of the complexity of the work – interventions need to happen at the top, the bottom and in the middle, strategically and at the coal-face, if system change is to occur.

General lessons

• Be aware of the challenge of partnership working – it is complicated and unpredictable, and often people are not able to speak for their organisation even though they have been selected as representatives.
• Stay in touch with service users, carers and the public, but be aware that they will lose interest if outcomes are not apparent.
• Be aware that local 'bottom up' priorities may be at odds with the national 'top down' policy agenda.
• Consider the risks involved in having only one project worker.
• You will inhabit a no man's land that exists in the spaces between services and their cultures. Find whatever support you can along the way!
• Resist the temptation to get involved with very specific service developments at an operational level, unless it has been clear all along that this is a potential outcome.
• Be realistic about timescales. Some experts estimate that whole system development takes 5–7 years.

Above all, accept that the eventual destination may not be at all as planned.

Conclusion: throwing stones or throwing birds?

In reflecting on our work we have begun to discover the utility of some of the ideas from complexity thinking. The biologist Richard Dawkins talks about the difference between throwing stones and throwing birds. When one throws stones, basic information about mass, velocity and trajectory is enough to make accurate predictions about where they will land and what sort of impact they will make. But when one throws birds one can be fairly sure that they will take off and at some point may land again. However, much of their behaviour will depend on many other variables and will not be easily predicted.

Historically, interventions in systems have tended to be conceived as stone throwing – so precise objectives are defined and clear outcomes expected. In fact it is still very much the case that strategic plans, and project outcomes alike are presented as predictable consequences of specific actions.

We are able to look back to the conceptual stage of the project and see the expectation that intervention A would result in B. The planning process for such initiatives demands that this sort of language is used.

In reality, as we have seen, many unforeseen factors impact on the trajectory of a chosen intervention, making it almost impossible to predict how a certain action or project will unfold. Significant personnel move on. Structures are dismantled. Project leaders get ill. Policies change. It is our experience that trying to create change in complex systems is more like throwing birds than stones. There were some very important outcomes but not necessarily those that were predicted.

'It has actually made people sit up and say "how can we do this better?" and "what can we do?" It has got the whole system seriously looking now at how they can contribute to a more co-ordinated approach.'

From Interim Evaluation Report

References

1   Department of Health (1998) *Modernising Mental Health Services: safe, sound and supportive*. DoH, London. www.doh.gov.uk

2   Pilgrim D and Rogers A (1993) Mental health service users' views of medical practitioners. *J Interprof Care*. **7**(2): 167–76.

3   Sainsbury Centre for Mental Health (2000) *Finding and Keeping: Review of recruitment and retention in the mental health workforce*. SCfMH, London.

4   Department of Health (1999) *National Service Framework for Mental Health (modern standards and service models)*. DoH, London.

5   Department of Health (2000) *The NHS Plan: A plan for investment, a plan for reform*. DoH, London.

6   Department of Health (2000) *A Health Service of all the Talents: developing the NHS workforce*. Consultation document on the review of workforce planning. DoH, London.

7   The Stationery Office (1999) *Saving Lives: Our healthier nation*. HMSO, London.

8   Kai J, Crosland A and Drinkwater C (2000) Prevalence of enduring and disabling mental illness in the inner city. *Br J Gen Pract*. **50**: 992–4.

9   Kendick T, Burns T, Freeling P and Sibbald B (1994) Provision of care to general practice patients with a disabling long term mental illness: a survey in 16 practices. *Br J Gen Pract*. **44**: 301–9.

10 Wilson K, Chen R, Taylor S, *et al.* (1999) Socio-economic deprivation and the prevalence and prediction of depression in older community residents: The MRC-ALPHA study. *Br J Psychiatry*. **175**: 549–53.

11. Weich S, Lewis G (1998) Poverty, unemployment and common mental disorders: population based cohort study. *BMJ*. **317**: 115–19.

12. Lewis G, Bebbington P, Brugha T, *et al.* (1998) Socioeconomic status, standard of living, and neurotic disorder. *Lancet.* **352**: 605–9.

13. Weich S and Lewis G (1998) Material standard of living, social class, and the prevalence of the common mental disorders in Great Britain. *J Epidemiol Community Health.* **52**(1): 8–14.

14. Driessen G, Gunther N and Van OS J (1998) Shared social environment and psychiatric disorder: multilevel analysis of individual and ecological effects. *Soc Psychiatry Psychiatr Epidemiol.* **33**(12): 606–12.

15   Kai J and Crosland A (2001) Perceptions of people with enduring mental ill health: a community-based study. *Br J Gen Pract.* **51**: 730–7.

Further reading

1   Plsek PE and Wilson T (2001) Complexity science: complexity, leadership and management in healthcare organisations. *BMJ.* **323**(7315): 746–9.

2   Pratt J, Gordon P and Plamping D (1999) *Working Whole Systems: putting theory into practice in organisations.* King's Fund, London.

3   Revans R (1998) *The ABC of Action Learning.* Lemos and Crane, London.

4   Wilson T, Holt T, Greehalgh T (2001) Complexity science: complexity and clinical care. *BMJ.* **323**(7314): 685–8.

CHAPTER 13

Responding to the needs of older people: a multidisciplinary community resource team approach

Ewan Dick and Claire Pinder

Differing and multiple needs

Consider this common situation:

> Mrs B is 84-years-old and had a stroke ten years ago with gradual deterioration in her functional ability ever since. Recently she has had a number of falls, lost confidence, and no longer feels able to socialise or get out to the shops. Isolation has slowly increased and affected her self-motivation. She also has early dementia. Her husband has arthritis and chronic obstructive airways disease and is dependent on her care. He is finding it difficult to understand changes in his wife. Tension is building between them. She will not countenance referral to social services...

Their GP, practice or community nurse is likely to already be involved. In responding, the usual pathways they might follow include:

- seeing a geriatrician for medical investigation of Mrs B's falls
- physiotherapy for assessment of possible functional problems contributing to her falls and improving her confidence when walking
- community occupational therapist to assess environmental causes of the falls and to address ways of maintaining safe, independent functioning

- psychogeriatrician assessment of cognitive decline and low mood
- the GP hoping they may be persuaded to accept home care services.

Too many cooks

Each of the above services will operate to their own criteria and waiting lists. They will be involved at different times, often working in isolation from one another. The clinicians, for example, will tend to focus on their own area of speciality. They may have little, if any, knowledge of the involvement or goals of other services, either now or previously. All this means lots of appointments and duplication of assessment, which is particularly unwelcome if you are already reluctant to accept referral or support from services.

Assessment out of context

Patients attending an outpatient clinic are out of context from their real life home setting. What may be unremarkable in a clinic looks very different at home. A clinician may not know that Mrs B has swapped her nightgown and slippers for a skirt and blouse for the first time in eight months to come to the clinic. Medication bottles presented in the consultation are one thing. Taking a look at the array of tablets scattered about the house is another. The odour in the home betrays the incontinence she denies in the clinic.

In fact, their only support is from their daughter who is now at breaking point. She has tried to persuade her mother to accept home care. She cannot continue to support them daily as well as doing their shopping, cooking, laundry and housework, on top of her own family's needs.

Elderly resource team

This chapter outlines an approach to supporting older people like Mr and Mrs B who commonly have complex needs in the community. The elderly resource team (ERT) is a multidisciplinary team working across the West of Newcastle upon Tyne. Awareness of the need for more comprehensive and co-ordinated assessment of older people, carried out within the community where older people live, has shaped development of the ERT. It offers an alternative to the traditional pathways of care above and to single professional assessment.

Local context and challenges

Newcastle PCT has 40 144 older people over the age of 65, with 42% of pensioners living alone. About half of this population live in the deprived West area including a significant proportion of minority ethnic groups.

While GP fundholding had led to patchy development of 'in-house' services for some, for example therapy, chiropody and social work staff, it was recognised that older people were not receiving co-ordinated services, often resulting in gradual, unmanaged deterioration. People with acute problems were not being supported at home. 'Inappropriate' hospital admissions were common. In addition, people in residential and nursing homes were not receiving equal services and support.

Birth of the resource team

A number of individuals contributed initially to the formation of the service, not least the developing roles of a community geriatrician and a community liaison nurse alongside a liaison GP from the locality. A primary care locality commissioning approach offered the flexibility to begin to address the perceived health and social needs of the local population, with resources initially identified as part of locality development funds devolved from the health authority.

Initially, the ERT comprised a community geriatrician, occupational therapist, chiropodist, physiotherapist, social worker and team assistant with administrative support and a team co-ordinator. As it has developed, the team has had support from an old age psychiatrist, dietician and liaison nurse in addressing the broad needs of service users.

Evidence base and rationale

There is considerable evidence that a multidisciplinary approach to patient care is often more effective.[1] In relation to older people in the community, with a breadth of health and social needs, this is even more appropriate.[2]

In the West area of Newcastle it was recognised that new service models needed to integrate both different professions and organisations. The aim was to develop a service across a locality area that responded to primary care teams, and bridged primary and secondary care, linking effectively with social services by co-ordinating and integrating relevant parts of existing services.

NSF for older people

The ERT approach pre-dated the subsequent NSF for Older People, which is now facilitating the more widespread development of multidisciplinary teams and intermediate care provision.

The National Service Framework for Older People (NSF for OP)[3] envisions a single assessment process (SAP). Subsequent guidance sets out that 'Local implementation of the SAP by health and social care systems will promote better care services and better outcomes for older people, and more effective use of professional resources. In particular, the SAP should ensure that the scale and depth of assessment are kept in proportion to older people's needs, agencies do not duplicate each other's assessments, and professionals contribute to assessments in the most effective way.'[4]

Although the ERT process emphasises screening, the four levels of assessment within the SAP are consistent with those used by the ERT. The team receive referrals ('contact'), following an 'overview' assessment, while the subsequent screening carried out by the team equates to a 'comprehensive' assessment, leading to the 'specialist' levels of assessment within the team.

Approach of the resource team

What would happen if Mrs B's GP referred her to the ERT? The referral can be classified urgent (response within two working days) or non-urgent (within two weeks). An ERT team member arranges a visit to carry out comprehensive screening (see below). This helps to identify Mrs B's needs and generates an agreed action plan, some issues requiring more urgent actions than others. For example, a medical assessment by the specialist geriatrician could be arranged within days via the local day hospital with findings fed back to the team to inform further interventions.

By co-ordinating input to clients the team can be sensitive with timing of visits, maintain effective communication, and minimise duplication through effective sharing of information. A weekly review meeting enables progress to be monitored and team members can offer their own experience and skills to influence the team approach to support the patient and their carers.

Mr and Mrs B are typical of those with a wide variety of problems and needs, which are inextricably linked. It is impossible to label their needs purely in social, medical, physical or mental health terms – they require a comprehensive multidisciplinary, multi-agency approach.

Development of the elderly resource team

Team members moved across the health and social care system to ensure the team effectively integrated with others. Many undertook joint posts resulting in close links with the local day hospital, geriatrician (by providing sessions with acute and rehabilitation wards), district nursing teams and the area social services team.

Early consultation was undertaken with providers, particularly targeting primary care teams, to identify key areas that the service would need to address. This enabled the team to identify relevant referral criteria, ensuring it was meeting the needs of the locality and its population.

Who are the clients?

The majority of people referred are frail and elderly, with an average age of 82 years. There are no restrictive age criteria in order to enable the potential referral of younger people, who can present with chronic degenerative conditions and equally complex needs that cannot be met by other specialist services.

A breakdown in support arrangements often prompts a referral to the team. Partners are likely to be elderly themselves and may be coping with their own health problems. Other family members find themselves in a caring role, which they feel unable or unwilling to fulfil. Other older people depend on informal support from friends and neighbours or formal support from social services, wardens or private arrangements. All of these can be challenged when increasing dependence occurs due to either physical or cognitive decline.

Reasons for referral to the team

Poor mobility and falls, or the risk of falls, are common reasons for referral. This is usually associated with difficulties around transfers and other activities of daily living. Other problems include unexplained deterioration, exacerbation or poor control of a chronic condition, an acute episode (e.g. urinary tract or chest infection) resulting in disorientation, inability to mobilise, or an acute event (e.g. transient ischaemic attack, stroke, myocardial infarction) where either the GP feels that the person does not require a hospital admission or the individual does not wish to be admitted. The team also has to be aware of other factors such as early signs of dementia, exacerbation of an established dementia, depression, social isolation and loss of motivation.

Screening and information gathering

The interdisciplinary team approach begins with a screening process. A multidisciplinary tool has been developed by the team that is used to identify client and carer needs and encompasses functional, physical, medical, social, mental health and carer issues.

Each team member has ongoing in-service training to gain a working knowledge of each other's roles and to understand each other's terminology. Thus all members are enabled to carry out screening of patients even though they will broach issues that will be outside their traditional clinical area. For example, a chiropodist exploring difficulties using cutlery or a social worker recording symptoms of dizziness.

From the screening process the team can identify an action plan and individual professionals will agree specific goals with the patient and the carer. There is no single pathway for intervention as each individual presents with unique needs.

Screening is supported by information given from other agencies that have previous or existing involvement. The information gathering process allows for appropriate referral to relevant professionals within the team and to other services such as community nursing, day hospital and old age psychiatry.

Co-ordination and communication

A key worker is identified to co-ordinate the team's involvement while joint notes are used to allow recording of detailed professional assessments and interventions as well as a running commentary of visits, actions, telephone calls, new information, case reviews, etc.

The 'communication page' is tested whenever information regarding our involvement is required. Any member of the team, including the administration staff, must be able to provide up-to-date and accurate information.

One of the major strengths of the ERT is that all staff are based together in a single office with comprehensive administrative support, which facilitates communication and planning.

All team members are managed by the ERT co-ordinator, which, for many, means someone outside their own profession. This central management model allows for clear lines of responsibility with a strategic overview of activity, performance and future opportunities for the service as well as the individuals within it. Professional supervision and support are clearly defined for all staff using clear professional structures (within the trust and social services) and each person has a responsibility to maintain these links.

The challenge of client centredness

Being truly client centred is a major challenge when setting realistic goals with vulnerable service users who have complex problems. It is possible to falsely raise expectations when entering into a critical situation where there are high levels of anxiety and stress, giving the impression that nothing is unachievable with such comprehensive support. It is also possible that skills on offer are turned down.

People do not live their lives expecting to find themselves relying on health and social services personnel to support them in old age. For many it is a threat to their independence. Team members find themselves negotiating with patients and carers, not enforcing services upon them. The team operates at their pace and with their permission. The picture of a passive, accepting, elderly person in a hospital bed, expecting to have procedures and assessments carried out on them, does not apply here.

Setting realistic goals

In order to set realistic goals, the limitations set by the patient's own physical and cognitive ability have to be recognised by team members as well as the individuals themselves. Limitations imposed by services also have to be realised – the intensity of physiotherapy input, the number of days available at the day centre or the ability of staff in a residential home to manage a fluctuating illness. Realistic goal setting has to take into account the needs and goals of the informal carers. These can often be in conflict with the needs and personal goals of the individual referred to the team.

The complexity and diversity of need presented by this group of older people mean that standard outcome measures cannot be easily applied. Significant changes or improvements in function or independence are not always expected, which emphasises the need for realistic, person-centred goals.

The duration of team involvement is tailored according to need (current average is 41 days). Avoiding caseload saturation requires careful management and is negotiated with primary and community care colleagues such as community nurses, GPs, community psychiatric nurses and social workers. With a client group who often have degenerative conditions and increasing frailty, these plans also have to take into account changing needs and possible referral back to ERT and/or other specialist services.

Challenging attitudes and the system

The developing team has, at times, had to challenge negative attitudes within 'the system'. These are not always explicit but may be systemic, historical, or based on misconceptions. For example, 'rehabilitation' is regularly used in relation to certain types of services for older people (usually therapy focused). However, when working with those with chronic or complex needs this term can detract from a realistic approach to intervention.

It is not uncommon for an older person to be identified as not having 'rehab potential', resulting in them effectively having therapeutic support withdrawn, and leaving the social worker to get on with finding a residential care home for long-term care.[5] The individual is not afforded every opportunity to continue living at home and goes into care unfulfilled in terms of achieving optimum functioning or with aspects of their lifestyle not being addressed in a therapeutic sense.

As a therapist there is often a perception that rehabilitation involves striving for distinct measurable physical achievements. However, in many cases a realistic intervention may not represent attaining significant improvements in physical function or independence, but rather may involve managing a deterioration, contributing to effective care planning and carer support, minimising risk and maximising quality of life for that individual.

Sustaining and developing workforce

These challenges have been tackled through supportive joint working rather than confrontation. By challenging the elements of the 'system' that are not flexible, it is possible to see the work as rewarding and enjoyable, requiring specialist support.

Different professional staff working within 'geriatric' services are not always seen as specialist. This is reinforced if staff do not have the opportunity or support to take risks and develop themselves or if their achievements are seen as minimal in a traditional 'rehab' sense.

The integrated and supportive team environment allows risks to be taken or for colleagues to be supported with difficult or potentially negative cases. We endeavour to extend this support to other primary and secondary care colleagues. Indeed, provision of external support by a specialist team such as the ERT may have long-term implications for how primary healthcare teams manage patients with complex problems, leading to more appropriate demands on the primary healthcare team.[6]

Wider learning

The ERT model has underlined positive messages about the feasibility and success of multi-agency working, the wider impact of health and social care and an awareness of the older person in society.

Beyond the locality, liaison nurses aligned to different PCTs are now linked with the ERT to facilitate greater links between primary care teams, residential and nursing homes and social services. These nurses, in conjunction with the team, have developed training and education opportunities for staff from residential and nursing homes and other community colleagues. Some of this training involves helping care staff, who are often professionally isolated, to explore and learn some principles of basic care and support of older people. However, there is also a facilitative element that brings together individuals across agencies to share and develop good practice through training sessions and workshops, and enables peer-support.

Conclusion: lessons for success

The elderly resource team has been built on locally driven and locally responsive processes. Key components for its success include the following.

- **Recognising, identifying and clarifying local need**: One model does not fit all. A locality approach to recognising need offers opportunities to analyse local health needs and begin to mould a service that meets those needs. The development of PCTs offers significant opportunity in this regard.
- **Joint working and multidisciplinary problem solving**: This is critical but the challenge of achieving it should not be underestimated. There has to be investment for longer-term benefits. Being based together, learning together, equity and collective responsibility all build a team.
- **Leadership, support and learning**: Clinicians do want to provide better services and work more efficiently. With leadership and support they will create systems and structures that enable this. A resource team of the type described needs time to become cohesive and share common ideals and focus. Each individual has to be confident and mature enough to allow their own professional boundaries to be challenged and to learn new skills and approaches.
- **Positive proactive care**: Establishing new ways of working does not

necessarily mean creating a new caseload for different professionals. Rather it involves working more efficiently with existing service users and proactively tackling problems and management in the community. A more positive and proactive model of care for older people is achievable. This is beneficial to clinicians but, most importantly of all, it is what older people and their families want.

References

1   Standing Medical advisery Committee (1990) *The Quality of Medical Care.* HMSO, London.

2   Stuck AE, Siv AL, Wieland GD and Adams J (1993) Comprehensive geriatric assessment – a meta-analysis of controlled trials. *Lancet.* **342**: 1032–6.

3   Department of Health (2001) *National Service Framework for Older People.* HMSO, London.

4   Department of Health (2002) *Single Assessment; Guidance for Local Implementation.* HMSO, London.

5   Audit Commission Briefing (2000) *The Way To Go Home.* The Audit Commission, London.

6   Robinson L and Drinkwater C (2000) Care of the frail elderly in the community: a critical incident study. *Primary Health Care Research and Development.* **1**: 163–77.

CHAPTER 14

Happy Hearts

Mary Robson

'Factors which make for health are concerned with a sense of personal and social identity, human worth, communication, participation in the making of political decisions, celebration and responsibility. The language of science alone is insufficient to describe health; the languages of story, myth and poetry also disclose its truth.'[1]

Community-based arts in health projects have sprung up across the UK since the late 1980s. The Happy Hearts Lantern in Wrekenton is one such event, bringing together arts, health, education and voluntary sector agencies to work at grass roots level to identify and address health needs. Here is its story.

In the mid 1990s the arts in health company Pioneer Projects was commissioned by Gateshead Council to produce a celebratory lantern procession with local people. It would be a finale event for Prime Time – a two year arts development programme for older people funded, amongst others, by the King's Fund.

As the project director designate, my first visit to Wrekenton was in the autumn, guided by Council Arts Officers. The view from Windy Nook, the aptly named local high spot, shows it to be surprisingly green given its unenviable and undeserved reputation as a 'blackspot'. The scar of the dismantled railway line divides the community into two – Springwell estate on one side and the rest of Wrekenton on the other. Nestled between are a clinic, a library and two primary schools.

At the time, Gateshead had the highest morbidity rate in coronary heart disease in England. Pioneer Project's previous work in the area had drawn on the image of the heart and established a good relationship with the local health promotion service. The health promotion mobile team was to be based in Wrekenton and so we decided to join forces. The artists would teach the health promotion personnel lantern making skills and share local contacts.

The common denominator between school, lantern workshop and health promotion bus is that each can induce wariness. To voluntarily step over the threshold into unfamiliar territory can be a daunting challenge – especially when there is a possibility of confirming an image of poor health and education. By holding the lantern workshops in the community rooms of Fell Dyke Primary School, and by including the health promotion personnel in the team, we made the whole experience informal and far less of a threat.

It was felt that the lantern parade should help banish the winter blues of February and herald the spring. The date was set for mid-March, just before British Summertime begins. The project was initially entitled 'Cold Hands, Warm Hearts'. Now, by popular demand from its participants, it is called Happy Hearts.

Teachers, health professionals and local artists learned how to make lanterns at an open day held a year previously for all interested parties. The project team attended Wrekenton network meetings – schools, churches, community education, social services, the youth service, libraries, health visitors and the police were all represented. From these meetings came more support for the project – St Oswald's Primary School and a girls group signed up to make images for the procession; a local computer group would produce the poster and the community policeman would organise the route and join us on the parade.

The Red Herring Bakery was commissioned to hold bread making workshops for Fell Dyke schoolchildren and their parents, and to build an outdoor brick oven at the school. This would be fired to bake bread made on the premises for the event. Soup is still made in a lot of homes in Wrekenton, we wanted to promote it further, and to have something delicious to dunk the bread into. Nursery children would be involved by making pictures with fresh fruit. A blacksmith made a steel framed heart to our design. Almost three metres high, it is the framework for the Heart of the Community Lantern.

The health promotion team initiated a lot of activities in the community room. Local women and school staff were happily plunged into aerobics, fitness training and healthy eating discussions. The strong relationships formed with the health promotion team, the support and mediation of the school staff and the Council Arts Officers plus a dose of pathological optimism from the participants made for a strong foundation for the first parade in March 1994.

The lanterns are made from withies – willow sticks – bound together with masking tape, covered in tissue paper and lit by candles. Two weeks of lantern workshops lead up to the procession. The community room became a 'congenial space', described below in an evaluation of the project:

'A congenial space consists of a spirit of high energy, laughter, purposeful and excited creative activity and the beginnings of trust, credibility and confidence. In a way, this space is a privileged ground between a community's potential for action and change and its alienated and deprived members. It is an embryonic focus for well being … It is also, hopefully, a space in which health and social workers can meet community members on their own terms.'[2]

A school class workshop would attract parents, some of whom had problems connecting with the school environment due to their less than happy experiences within the education system. Slowly, a gang of women and the occasional man became involved. No longer threatened, the power of chat became the conduit for discussion – sometimes serious, at other times hysterical – of health, life and death. At the centre of it all was the art and activity of lantern making. Parents would come to help their child make one and would still be coming days after that one had been finished. From simple materials appeared magical objects. Soup was made every day for lunch. Eating together became an important focus for the team and the regulars that continues to this day.

Two hundred people turned up on the cold and damp evening of 18 March. When all the lanterns were lit, the band began to play and off we went. As dusk fell, the lanterns changed from white lumpen shapes into delicate lacy structures, glowing amber, bobbing along on an incoming tide of darkness. Each individual effort found its place in the collective stream: none was dispensable. The streets of Wrekenton at night were suddenly transformed.

At the end of the evening, The Heart of the Community was placed on the top of the hill behind Fell Dyke School. Fireworks burst over and around it and finished with the heart glowing red. It has proved a lasting and potent image. A teacher's husband, recovering from a heart attack commented:

'Seeing that big heart light up made my heart feel better.'

Back inside the community room for bread, soup and fruit after the fireworks, the then deputy head of Fell Dyke School said to me:

'When you came here and said "We're all going to make lanterns out of sticks and glue and walk down the streets with them", well, I thought you were mad. I'd never have believed what I've seen tonight. Look, it's Friday night in Wrekenton and everybody's eating brown bread and soup – and enjoying it.'

March 2000 saw the seventh lantern procession. Over the intervening years, it has become a traditional event. Developments have occurred that could not have been planned. Every lantern has the image of a heart in it and lanterns are often made in memory of those who have died and for those newly born. Children feel able to disclose and discuss their innermost thoughts and feelings in a lantern workshop. As a result, local women have asked for training to help with child protection issues locally. An emotional literacy initiative founded by Happy Hearts and the local public health promotion team has begun in both schools – preparing pupils for the transition to secondary education.

Food is a continuing theme. As well as bread and soup making, communal eating has become a feature of lantern workshops, facilitating discussions about healthy eating and adding to the welcoming and relaxed atmosphere. Children are offered prepared fruit as a gift as part of their lantern experience. For many it is their first taste of melon or strawberry. Coming back after school to complete their lantern, they invariably ask for a piece of fruit to keep them going until tea time.

A connection with the Shiatsu College in Gateshead means that massage has become available for participants and professionals. One year there was also reflexology, which proved an unexpected success with school staff as a 'stressbuster'. Staff from both primary schools use the event as the focus for their health curriculum activities and have consistently gained healthy school awards.

Local people have formed The Happy Hearts Alliance to help fundraise and keep the spirit of the project going throughout the year. Members have spoken at conferences and gatherings and are now actively involved in other arts in health initiatives. Young people who have been involved since they were seven years old have become apprentices to the project. Their secondary school headteacher has encouraged their involvement. They have followed their elders by banding together as The Young Hearts. As well as fundraising, they are working with artists and health professionals to develop projects outside Wrekenton. Since 2000, they have run workshops and demonstrations in Northumberland and Sunderland. Plans are afoot for Happy Hearts 2003 to be host to a contingent from Hendon. They want a lantern event there and are partnering local people in Wrekenton for help and advice.

Happy Hearts contributed to the local community carnival for the first time in 1999. The Heart of the Community was taken out for a daylight appearance, surrounded by processional imagery created by schoolchildren, The Young Hearts and Mothers and Toddlers.

The same group went for organised walks that year – both on an art trail along the newly developed quayside in Newcastle and around the estates in Wrekenton. Comparing and contrasting the two resulted in a map – an artwork encapsulating the needs of the residents and illustrating how

Wrekenton could be a healthier neighbourhood. As a planning tool, it has fed into the evaluation of the project by the King's Fund. The resultant long-term goal of all involved was to have a permanent home for Happy Hearts. First choice was the site of the soon to be demolished school hall. Although felt by many to be the home of the project – where it was born and where it belongs – we have had to let that notion go, as a private developer has bought the land and has plans to build houses there. The building we dream of will be environmentally sensitive, with a large hall and residential accommodation. The kitchens and community café will be supported by a big garden.

Until the dream comes true, securing venues for the workshops and the finale will continue to prove troublesome. The Fell Dyke School site seemed the perfect venue – as well as the hill it had the large detached hall, the biggest in the area. Its demolition this year has meant that the finale has to be completely rethought. The potential replacement of a local Methodist hall had to be turned down because the church elders would not allow Shiatsu massage to take place there. The local secondary school gym was tried as an alternative a couple of years ago, but it proved impossible to add an outdoor fireworks element to the evening. Having to bring the big heart indoors meant a different atmosphere. Whilst it looked impressive as part of a large tableau, something of the potency of the image was lost. It needs to be seen from a distance, as part of the landscape under a night sky. Indoors, it was always a lantern. Outdoors, it is the Heart of the Community.

Maintaining the Happy Hearts Alliance and the Young Hearts groups is a sensitive task that falls outwith the more obvious job description of the project workers. Without the input and encouragement of the professional team, fundraising and development at a local level would not happen. Delicate mediation is required in the midst of a minefield of interpersonal relationships and is never to be underestimated. This means being involved at every stage, together with the participants, without regard to time and motion. It takes a long time but is never onerous. It can seem frighteningly unfocused and informal at times but maintains a vibrancy within a frame-work of trust and respect that counters any leanings towards the institutional.

Happy Hearts now directly involves up to 500 people. It continues to develop, spawning activities that will take place throughout the year. It is no longer simply an annual lantern procession, yet that remains its central focus. It reflects a growing school of thought that good relationships are a major determinant of health. All involved feel that the strong, collective and good time nature of the event feeds individual and communal health needs. Indeed, it is now a very particular tradition. Ali Magee, a participant from the very beginning, put it like this:

'In Wrekenton, there's Christmas and there's lanterns ... It's definitely made me think about my health and my kid's health, and given me the confidence to do something about it – we can choose to be healthier.'

References

1   Wilson M (1975) *Health is for People*. Darton, Longman and Todd, London.

2   Angus J and Murray F (2002) *An Enquiry Concerning Possible Methods for Evaluating Arts for Health Projects*. Community Health UK (1999), re-issued CAHHM.

CHAPTER 15

Facilitating work, social support and health in an ethnically diverse community

Joe Kai, Billy Foreman, Bhavna Solanki &
Shagufta Khan

Introduction

Nasim Ahmed's doctor says her son, who is almost 2-years-old, needs iron. The GP has given her some syrup and told her to give the boy more fruit, meat and vegetables. Nasim left the surgery worried and puzzled: her boy ate perfectly well – he had lots of meat and he seemed well. What was wrong with her son? Was it serious? Was this something to do with her husband's diabetes? They weren't sure about that either and her husband had now lost his job because his sight had failed. Nasim wants to do her best for her family's health, but she has neither much money nor ready sources of practical help and advice.

Nasim is not her real name but she lives in Sparkbrook, an inner city area of Birmingham where 60% of the population is South Asian, predominantly from Pakistani Muslim communities. Stories like this tell of a local demography laden with persistently poor health, educational, environmental and economic indices. For example, the perinatal mortality rate here was 14.6 per 1000 live births between 1989 and 1993 – the highest in the city and twice the national average.

Sparkbrook Community Parents scheme was developed as a response to poor health outcomes, but also as a way of bringing together local health and community services with the wider world of economic opportunity and urban regeneration. This article outlines the initiative's formative experiences four years on.

Opportunities and contexts

There has been increasing recognition of inequality of access to appropriate health services for many people from minority ethnic communities.[1] In Birmingham, minority ethnic communities form a quarter of the population, but there is a long way to go before staff mix across health and other services will reflect that diversity. Such development in primary and community care is a major issue given their critical role as points of access to the NHS and other services.[2]

In Sparkbrook, local people with some part time training were raising awareness about health issues in their communities as 'lay health advisers'. However, they worked as volunteers and opportunities for their further training and employment were lacking. At the same time in the late 1990s Birmingham Health Authority and City Council were developing family support projects across the city focusing upon poverty and inequality. Yet regeneration programmes were delivering little to women and minority communities.[3] There was now a major opportunity to act by using local regeneration funding and the European Social Fund (ESF). The aim was to train local people, particularly those from ethnic minority communities, to develop new skills for health and social care services, and for their employment in supporting families affected by what is now called social 'exclusion'.

The case for social support

The value of social support is increasingly recognised. Social support is concerned with the practical and emotional components of caring, advice, information and help rather than 'clinical care'.[4] For example, such support creates better physical and emotional health for women and their children, in particular for those living in poor material circumstances.[5,6]

The Sparkbrook scheme has been influenced by family support initiatives in the US and the Netherlands,[7] Dublin,[8] France, Italy and elsewhere. For example, in the US dramatic reductions in infant mortality among disadvantaged communities have been achieved.[7,9]

Local recruitment of people to deliver support within their own communities also appears to yield longer-term outcomes, for example mothers may be more likely to go back into education, and on to paid employment, and children may experience better nutrition, fewer accidents, and less morbidity.[8] While Sparkbrook 'community parents' have engaged local women as a starting point, they have not focused solely upon maternal and child health. Rather, they have been identifying needs and realistic opportunities with women in pursuit of the broader health aspirations of local families.

Securing creative partnerships and funding

The development and funding of the scheme have been built upon partnerships. Initially, Birmingham Voluntary Services Council acted as the scheme's accountable non-public body for the ESF, while the then Southern Birmingham Community NHS Trust (SBCT) administered support to the community parents during their training and development. Birmingham Health Authority (BHA) provided the momentum for the partnership and supported part of community parent salaries. Together with the social services department, these partners facilitated a 'market' for the employment of community parents in health and social care settings. In concert, Joseph Chamberlain College (JCC) and later South Birmingham College developed the training and accreditation of the community parents. A training and placements officer was initially employed by SBCT (now South Birmingham PCT) to secure community placements in collaboration with other partners.

In starting, just over half of scheme funding came from mainstream resources, with the remainder from the European Communities employment (INTEGRA) programme of the ESF. Local regeneration money (SRB II) then matched this funding for subsequent years. Traditional boundaries needed to be challenged to create the funding opportunity. For example, in the absence of an established market place for employment, the DfEE needed to be persuaded that the scheme would indeed be a legitimate use of the ESF. The scheme argued it was *making a market* by creating new roles to meet previously unmet needs.

Getting started

Local interest in becoming a community parent was generated by word of mouth, existing lay and family support networks and, most successfully, by approaching women through local primary schools. This demanded patience and sensitivity to women's apprehensions about full time college training, and concerns about how further education and status might potentially be perceived within some families. A lot of time was invested in seeking women who were motivated and enthusiastic. A founding cohort of 20 women –

mainly from Pakistani but including Sikh and Indian communities – were recruited after written application and interview in 1998. They were aged between 18 and 48. Some had graduate qualifications from their home country, but most had secondary school level education to aged 16 or below. None of the women were in paid employment and most were parents with child care commitments.

Realistic support for women

The women were supported financially during training in recognition of the skills they already had and their potential contribution in the future. During academic terms they received a weekly allowance (£127) and further support if registered child care was sought (nursery or childminder) of up to £100 per week per child. This was a major attraction and indeed prerequisite for most women. However, it created practical problems. Six women originally recruited dropped out before the course commenced because this extra financial support would push them in to the 'benefits trap'. They would have forfeited their entitlement to certain welfare benefits, e.g. housing, council tax and school dinner benefits, and be worse off materially as a result. For some of the first group of 20 women who ultimately did do the course, this issue remained a burden. Although they were no worse off during term times, during holidays they received no training allowance and became re-entitled to welfare benefits – however, bureaucratic delays and inflexibility resulted in these not being paid. A further tension was that for some women whose children would be looked after by extended family, course attendance was only feasible if they could still attract the financial support for child care.

Community parents' training

The first group of women trainees engaged in a year of full-time training, involving three days a week at college and two days a week in supervised placements in the community. They worked towards obtaining a combination of Level 2 National Vocational Qualification (NVQ) and a BTEC National Diploma (in Early Years: Care and Education). Development of their training required innovation and creativity on the part of college tutors and the scheme's training and placements officer. For example, learning needed to be community-focused and culturally relevant. Workshops for trainees led by local professionals and voluntary agencies were facilitated that ranged, for example, from giving advice about welfare rights and benefits, debt counselling and equal opportunities through to learning about nutrition, pregnancy and breast feeding, child protection, genetic disorders and haemoglobinopathies. This diverse and practical orientation of training has proved vital.

There was a particular emphasis upon supervised placements given that accreditation based solely on traditional NVQ modules did not deliver the necessary knowledge or flexibility for learning and working. Examples of community attachments included work with health visitors and GP surgeries (e.g. befriending mothers in baby clinics); local voluntary agency run/social services linked family centres; parent partnership projects in primary schools; housing agencies and Asian women's refuge centres.

Women's education and training were formally accredited not only for their envisaged new roles but in order to provide them with pathways into further training and education opportunities and thus access to employment opportunities in health and social care. Such approaches are potentially challenging but similar experiences elsewhere have been encouraging.[10] The first cohort of 20 women successfully completed this training in 1999. Subsequent cohorts of 20 women each year have increasingly included women from African Caribbean, and also Irish and Chinese, communities, but difficulty recruiting those from Bangladeshi communities remains an issue.

Birth of a community business

By 2001, 18 of the first cohort of women and 7 of the second cohort had gained employment within a month of finishing their course. One of the requirements of the ESF sponsor is that beneficiaries cannot be directly employed by the public sector. In order to negotiate this, and to provide a supportive and community-focused structure for the women, all have been employed by a new community business, 'Compare'. This is a company limited by guarantee with a board of directors mainly comprising people already involved with the development of the scheme. The community business then contracts with other agencies, including public agencies. Importantly, employers were encouraged and supported to develop new roles for the community parents by receiving a substantial proportion of salaries (50%, then 30%, then 25%) in the first three years of the scheme from the then BHA. Subsequently, Compare has promoted the role of community parents to successfully attract contracts from agencies.

New roles in the community

The women are now working in a range of environments. For example, some are being employed by local PCTs and are based in health centres.

Returning to families like Nasim's, the community parents are working with health visitors and nurses to address pressing public health issues for local minority ethnic communities, such as anaemia in children, dental health and diabetes, by providing practical help, advice and explanation to mothers and families. There have inevitably been some challenges in terms of their overlap and perceived status in relation to existing bilingual linkworker colleagues. Primary care workers have also more easily seen the advantages of bilingual communication alone while neglecting the expertise and knowledge of community parents. As their new 'paraprofessional' roles and relationships develop and become seen as complementary to the roles of others, such tensions may be negotiated but they, perhaps predictably, remain a challenge to the differing professional hegemonies.

Other women are engaging parents in local primary schools, e.g. supporting health awareness, ESOL and computer training classes. Some of the community parents are working in social services linked family centres, e.g. providing social support for vulnerable and recently immigrated families. Some women have gone on to higher education opportunities and other employment. For example, one has become an outreach worker for a local Sure Start initiative in an area with an expanding South Asian population and is providing parenting support and information to families.

A key aim is trying to build up self-confidence and skills in people who are at risk of being overwhelmed by the overburdened circumstances in which they live, so that they stand a better chance of maintaining their health and well being. Work is also oriented toward advocacy, confronting rights and barriers rather than a more traditional approach to inequality of access to services that centres upon issues of language, e.g. interpreters and translated material. The latter may have little impact upon access to, and appropriateness of, services if the communities concerned do not assume their right to the service or indeed have not experienced that assumption. The community parents are seeking to create a shared community presumption that local services exist to meet *their* needs.

Mobilising faith communities

Work in Birmingham has demonstrated that, given the opportunity, faith communities are keen to engage with opportunities to improve their health. Complementing the community parents scheme, a male Muslim development worker has been appointed within another family support initiative, to work with men and develop sessions held in local mosques. These include discussion of specific priorities such as postnatal depression in women and prostate cancer, in addition to general men's health issues. He is raising awareness of health concerns among local communities in relation to children's health, through faith based supplementary school activities. For example, local evidence of very poor public dental health in children has led to developing appropriate curriculum options to integrate public health messages into mainstream education in local primary schools.

Early experiences of community parents

Many community parents came to the scheme with a considerable range of skills and potentials that they have been able to better realise through their new roles. For others the scheme has been more readily empowering and has raised their confidence and self-esteem. The training was enjoyable but hard. Women faced challenges negotiating their commitment to the course, assignments and work with their family and child care. However, many have appreciated being able to manage their own learning independently. Here, the opportunity for regular feedback and debriefing sessions during their training was particularly helpful. Subsequently, becoming part of the community business has been important in providing security of employment. It has offered community parents valuable support outwith their employed environment and women have been encouraged to organise and have representation that could speak for them as a group. Some experiences of the community parents are relayed below.

Case examples

'A' is an Indian woman with two young children who heard of the scheme through her daughter's school. The opportunity to gain qualifications beyond her existing GCSEs and to receive an allowance and support for child care were significant incentives. She recalls having to think on her feet when asked how she would respond to a hypothetical situation at interview, before being surprised by how 'in-depth' – both theoretically and practically – the course had been. In her community placement she was able to make use of skills she had hereto had no opportunity to use – initiating free computing and ESOL classes for South Asian parents in a local primary school while their children were in class.

'B' had obtained a psychology degree in Pakistan before coming to England where she married and became a mother. The scheme offered her the opportunity to build upon her education and obtain health-related work.

In contrast, 'C' had little formal educational attainments and had spent most of the past 18 years raising her children before joining the course. She found the assignments difficult, particularly as she had never used a computer before and had to write them by hand initially.

'D' says the scheme has helped her move forward from a position of no confidence and isolation as a young mother to one where she is now supporting women in considerable distress in local hostels, and has developed a network of new friends and colleagues. She wants to go on to train as a social worker.

E's training is helping her disseminate health messages in ways previously unavailable to local people. She can use her familiarity with local cultural contexts and beliefs to deconstruct myths or fears about health issues, and as a community member feel trusted by others. She gives an example of setting up a session about diabetes in a local school, resourced by a dietician and health visitor. Word spread, and attendance exceeded expectations with 21 women coming to learn about diabetes and its management in relation to Asian diets. She feels strongly that this sort of overture to her community can engage and influence the broad health of households rather than just individual mothers or children.

Toward the future

In sustaining the momentum of the scheme, the training programme is now being offered as a mainstream college option and is evolving from a BTEC focused upon 'early years care' to a broader care diploma. Thus, a wider constituency of learners may gain from this training, which may then become reflected in career choices and practices to the benefit of disadvantaged and minority ethnic communities. However, training of women has posed challenges for the educational institutions involved in terms of supporting some with no previous formal qualifications. Recruitment for training has needed to be targeted more closely to match the later requirements of job roles.

As initial ESF support has diminished, the weekly allowance to trainees has unfortunately had to be reduced although this has meant that trainees avoid the 'benefits trap'. It remains to be seen if this will still enable all women from different backgrounds and circumstances to participate, and if financial support to employers will be successful in allowing new posts to be established. Other challenges remain, such as engaging more women from Bangladeshi communities, and the evolution of new relationships with other professionals as community parent roles develop.

Crucially, the scheme has been adequately resourced beyond the short term. Continuing SRB and ESF funding for the scheme has been focused more directly in subsequent years upon certain public health issues – perinatal mortality, low birthweight and disability. This will create opportunities for further training for community parents and will extend their current roles.

The new community business is attempting to ensure a locally sustainable and managed infrastructure that retains a community focus. The advantage it confers is the support of women who may be at risk of exploitation by other professionals unclear about roles and remits. A tension is the need to evolve new roles in different agencies that genuinely address gaps in access to and provision of services rather than roles that speak only to existing professionals' agendas. Key challenges for the community business are sustaining structures and processes that maintain the involvement and voice of community parents themselves at decision-making board level. Secondly, there is a need to resist 'holding on' to its employees at the expense of encouraging their development and entry into the mainstream market for employment.

In conclusion, the initial objectives of the scheme have been met. Women from local communities have graduated through training when opportunities of this kind have not previously been available to them. They are now being employed to improve access to formal and informal care, and are developing support for health with respect to local community contexts. Many women have found the going tough but have endured and have felt empowered. Others have succeeded when they have conventionally been stereotyped as women whose cultural values would preclude them developing careers. Here the support that many women have received from their partners and families has indeed given the lie to others' assumptions.

References

1   Smaje C (1995) *Heath, Race and Ethnicity: Making sense of the evidence*. King's Fund, London.

2   Kai J (1999) Valuing ethnic diversity in primary care. *Br J Gen Pract*. **49**: 171–3.

3   Riseborough M (1997) *The Gender Report: women and regional regeneration in the Midlands*. A report of SRB III bids in the region. University of Birmingham, Birmingham.

4   Oakley A (1992) *Social Support and Motherhood*. Blackwell, Oxford.

5   Benzeval M, Judge K and Whitehead M (1995) *Tackling Inequalities in Health: an agenda for action*. King's Fund, London.

6   Spencer B, Thomas H and Morris J (1989) A randomised controlled trial of the provision of a social support service during pregnancy: The South Manchester Family Worker Project. *BJOG*. **96**: 281–8.

7   Hanrahan M and Prinsen B (1997) *Community Health, Community Care, Community Support*. Netherlands Institute for Care and Welfare, Mothers Inform Mothers Co-operative and the Bernard van Leer Foundation, Utrecht.

8   Johnson Z, Howell F and Molloy B (1993) Community mothers programme: randomised controlled trial of non-professional intervention in parenting. *BMJ*. **306**: 1449–552.

9   McFarlane J (1996) De madres a madres: an access model for primary care. *Am J Public Health*. **86**: 879–80.

10   Kai J and Hedges C (1999) Minority ethnic community participation in needs assessment and service development in primary care: perceptions of Pakistani and Bangladeshi people about psychological distress. *Health Expectations*. **2**: 7–20.

CHAPTER 16

A primary care clinic for drug dependence: addressing the heroin problem in Sheffield

Jenny Keen, Martin Bennett and Mick Down

Introduction

Drug misuse and addiction are inextricably linked to deprivation and poverty. Heroin addiction affects around 1% of adults in inner cities.[1] It brings with it a multitude of other problems: crime to finance the heroin habit, commonly with accompanying prostitution and imprisonment;[2] problems for the children of addicted individuals whose parents are often absent, intoxicated, or imprisoned;[3] poor health for the individuals themselves with high mortality, and drug related morbidity such as deep vein thrombosis, septicaemia and overdose, transmission of blood-borne viruses by sharing of injection equipment, and poor functioning with exclusion from employment.[4]

Like other cities[5,6] and following national guidance,[7,8] Sheffield has looked to primary care to develop services for heroin users. This chapter describes a new primary care-based intermediate level service.

Accessing services

Healthcare of heroin users has long been neglected in medical training, with GPs feeling inadequately trained to manage needs. Indeed, some GPs have historically been unwilling to offer any services to heroin users[9,10] with debate about whether substitute opiates should even be prescribed in primary care.[11]

Many drug users perceive GPs as uninterested and unhelpful. This is compounded when some drug users, often desperate for treatment, have behaved in a disruptive way in GP surgeries and elsewhere. Meanwhile, in Sheffield as elsewhere, secondary care services have been in danger of being swamped by the demand for treatment.

Recent guidance,[12] recognising training as key, suggests that all doctors should be competent to deal with drug related problems and that the number of doctors treating drug users in primary care in a shared care framework should be increased. Training has recently been introduced by the Royal College of General Practitioners.

Harm minimisation

Harm minimisation[13] focuses on reducing the risk of drug misuse to the individual and to society. This is often by provision of replacement opiate prescribing, without in all cases aiming specifically at a 'cure' for the individual's drug problem. The concept of harm minimisation has led to the development of a 'hierarchy' of goals of drug treatment.[14,15]

The rationale is the chronic relapsing nature of heroin addiction, which means that total abstinence for long-term users is often hard to achieve. Good evidence indicates a harm minimisation approach – methadone maintenance in particular – reduces the risks of illicit drug use,[4,5,16] reducing crime[17] and improving quality of life.[18]

Local context

In the 1990s there was increasing pressure on the existing under-funded specialist substance misuse service with waiting lists in excess of two years for maintenance treatment in Sheffield. Drug-related deaths were rising. Only a few local GP practices were prepared to prescribe methadone for heroin users and they had rapidly become swamped, developing waiting lists themselves. Inappropriate prescribing of benzodiazepines and dihydrocodeine for drug users was also occurring.

Drug users accessing treatment were confined to those prioritised, for example because of pregnancy or willingness to accept a short-term treatment such as lofexidine detoxification. There was no realistic option for GPs wishing to refer patients for medium to long-term methadone prescribing.

Getting support to move forward

Nationally, health authorities had been asked to prioritise services for drug users and develop primary care responses.[7,8] In Sheffield a coalition of individuals from various agencies, including a large centrally located pharmacy, worked with Sheffield Health Authority on a service specification for a new primary care-led clinic. The result was the development of a new primary care clinic for drug dependence, which opened in April 1999. The initiative was funded by the health authority and was endorsed by the local medical committee.

Developing the project

Rationale

It was acknowledged that achieving a position where the majority of GPs managed the drug misuse related treatment of their own drug using patients was likely to be slow. The idea of the clinic was that it would act on a deputising basis for GPs who were not ready to undertake their own prescribing, in a similar way that the GP out of hours co-operative worked. Prescribing and management of the drug problem would be undertaken by the clinic but the prescribing costs would be charged to the prescribing budget of the GP with whom the patient was registered. The clinic would be based in a 'provider' organisation, Community Health Sheffield, but funded directly from the waiting list initiative and drug development monies of Sheffield Health Authority. With the move to PCTs, the North Sheffield PCT took over as host organisation and the Drug Action Team took over the commissioning role.

Philosophy of the clinic

Harm minimisation (see above) rather than abstinence from all drugs was to be the primary aim of the clinic, although patients wishing to work towards abstinence were encouraged. The chronic relapsing nature of heroin addiction was recognised in the clinic protocol.

This required the support of committed individuals as the funding organisations were under financial pressure to find 'quick fix' solutions to 'cure' people of drug dependence.

The service

Long-term maintenance prescribing was provided for the majority of patients at the outset, although more recently the full range of community treatment options was made available. To encourage GPs to undertake their own prescribing, a quick turnaround scheme was set up: GPs could get a patient seen very quickly, stabilised in the clinic and then returned to their care after three months. The clinic did not take on patients for long-term treatment who were already on successful methadone maintenance with their GPs.

The prescribing of methadone by GPs outside the clinic was encouraged from the outset, with clinic staff becoming involved in developing local clinical governance guidance. Where possible, clinic staff contacted GPs in cases where the patient was completely stable and heroin free and where the patient was being seen six to eight weekly on a routine stable maintenance dose. GPs were asked to take over the long-term prescribing with the clinic taking back patients if they should relapse into instability.

A further role was to contribute to the development of training for GPs and other health service professionals and to contribute to further development of primary care treatment of drug users in the city.

Staffing and organisation

The clinic started with six doctor sessions, a full-time clinical nurse specialist, a half-time manager and one clerical officer. At the end of the first year, 200 patients were in treatment. By 2003 staffing had increased to 18 doctor sessions, two full-time nurses, a full-time manager and four clerical staff with two seconded drugs workers and 550 patients. The core budget for the clinic has remained small and it continues to cost less than £700 per year to treat a patient within the service, excluding pharmacy costs. Waiting times have remained consistently short.

The pharmacy network

Community pharmacists in Sheffield have always been involved in treatment of drug users. They have also been targets for drug-related crime ranging from forged prescriptions via shop lifting and burglary to armed robbery. Consequently, in a similar stance to other healthcare professionals, many were unenthusiastic about offering services to drug users. Despite this, the first pharmacy-based needle exchange scheme is thought to have started in Sheffield in 1988 and by the early 90s quite a well developed system involving 15 community pharmacies was in place. Over the next few years there was recognition of the need for supervised methadone consumption and a number of pharmacies agreed to undertake this task on an individual basis as no funding was available.

At the time of the development of the Primary Care Clinic for Drug Dependence, the majority of supervised dispensing and administration of methadone was undertaken by one centrally located pharmacy. The Local Pharmaceutical Committee and the health authority jointly developed a service specification for a comprehensive pharmacy service for substance misusers, embracing support for all clients receiving prescribed treatment and including supervised administration, monitoring of treatment progress, harm minimisation advice and, later, direct referral for untreated patients.

Following a tendering process, a contract to manage community pharmacy services for drug misusers was awarded to the central pharmacy (Associated Chemists (Wicker) Ltd), but conditional on a network of participating pharmacies being recruited to the scheme. The managing pharmacy successfully recruited other pharmacies in the city so that patients could elect to receive initial supplies through the central pharmacy or a more local pharmacy. The contract for the pharmacy-based services included separate funding for the management of the scheme and also included management of the local pharmacy-based syringe and needle scheme.

The scheme was a hub and spoke model open to all pharmacies in the city. To encourage participation, Associated Chemists, the hub pharmacy, agreed to undertake daily supervised supply during the patient's 'stabilisation' period, after which, with agreement, the patient could be transferred to a local participating pharmacy of their choice. The local pharmacist would be assured that, should any problems arise, the patient could be transferred back to the central hub pharmacy. Registration involves other obligations on the pharmacy concerned such as close liaison with prescribers over missed doses and the health of the patient, registering each patient on the scheme, accepting back used needles and syringes, timely return of forms, etc. The hub pharmacy provides back up in a number of ways including administering the scheme, supplying various forms and files, paying the pharmacy and the provision of monthly statistics. This degree of support enabled 46 of Sheffield's 105 pharmacies (44%) to register and take part in the scheme by 2003.

Close co-operation between pharmacies and the clinic was essential to maintain exchange of information about prescriptions and the well being of patients. Data on non-collection of prescriptions proved invaluable in monitoring whether, for instance, patients had gone into custody or hospital or for some other reason were not taking their treatment. This was an important safeguard for prescribers and patients alike.

The pharmacy scheme has been a success with pharmacists, prescribers and patients and has been essential to the development of the primary care service.

Evidence-based protocol

Available research evidence and national guidelines[12] were used to optimise safety and provide a template for GPs wishing to start prescribing.

In order to practise the optimal harm minimisation protocol, the clinical protocols in Box 16.1 were agreed.

Box 16.1: Clinical protocols

- All patients are started on daily supervised consumption of replacement medication at a named local chemist.
- Methadone mixture 1mg/ml, lofexidine, naltrexone and buprenorphine (Subutex) are the mainstay of treatment.
- Injectables are not prescribed and tablets are prescribed only in exceptional circumstances.
- Benzodiazepines are not prescribed except in the case of patients stabilised on and dependent on prescribed benzodiazapines, in which case reducing regimens are started.
- Dihydrocodeine, which is not licensed for the treatment of drug dependence, is not prescribed.
- There is no upper limit on dosage and it was noted that programmes employing higher dosages tend to have better results.[19]
- Patients are not expelled from the programme for failure to comply with treatment (i.e. use of illicit drugs) but they are expelled from the programme for dishonest acts such as prescription forgery. It was noted that studies had shown retention in treatment as an important marker for successful patient outcomes.[20]
- Patients remain on daily supervised consumption until stability has been achieved.
- Harm minimisation is the primary aim of the clinic rather than abstinence, but patient goals and progress are reviewed three monthly.
- Patients receive support when required both from the clinic staff and from local voluntary agencies.
- Close co-ordination and co-operation between clinic, pharmacies and GPs are central to the service.
- Patients who are pregnant, have serious psychiatric co-morbidity or are under 18, and those who exclusively use stimulant drugs, are referred on to the specialist service.

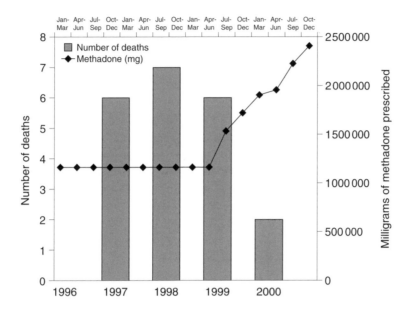

Figure 16.1 Numbers of methadone deaths in Sheffield 1997–2000.

Figure 16.1 shows the number of deaths considered by the Sheffield Coroner to have been caused by methadone, and mg of methadone dispensed in the city, with estimated maximum figures before 1999. Between 1999 and 2000 methadone deaths fell from six to two in spite of the fact that the quantity of methadone dispensed in the city had more than doubled during this time.

Outcomes of clinic after one year

After one year there were 200 patients in treatment, eliminating the former waiting list. In spite of the maintenance orientation of the clinic 13 patients had been discharged drug free. Approximately 15% of all referrals had been made under the quick turnaround arrangement with patients taken back by their GPs for long-term prescribing. A number of other GPs had agreed to take long-term stable patients back into their care when they had not originally planned to do so.

Outcomes for patients – risk-taking behaviour, consumption of illicit drugs (with urinalysis) and criminal activity (from criminal records) were formally measured throughout the first year by an independently funded research study.[21] As in other primary care-based studies[5,22] findings show highly significant reductions in risk-taking behaviours, consumption of heroin and criminal conviction rates, alongside significant improvements in physical and mental health and social functioning of the patients.

Individual Patient Outcomes

After one year or less in treatment many patients were in visibly better health having gained many pounds in weight and improving their overall level of nutrition and self care. Patients themselves attributed these improvements to no longer having to commit criminal acts or spend £50 to £100 a day on their addiction.

Many felt liberated by being allowed to stabilise on a dose of methadone and not being automatically expected to reduce it. Many had experienced treatment where there was an upper limit put on the amount of daily methadone, which had never allowed them to stop using heroin, because it had never been enough to abolish withdrawal symptoms.

The system of supervised consumption, at least in the initial stages, meant that the clinicians felt free to prescribe as much methadone as the patient required without fearing that this would be diverted to the black market. In spite of this control, the clinic experienced an extremely low drop out rate as compared with other services.[4,16,23]

Among the most satisfactory outcomes were those of the older patients, often with children, who had struggled with their heroin problem for years and for whom abstinence-based treatment had been tried and failed. Many rapidly became very stable, stating at the outset that they only needed a regular methadone prescription in order to stabilise and in general they coped with this very well. The probable benefits for their children are the subject of further research.

Drug related deaths in the city

Prior to the clinic opening, methadone-related deaths in the city had been rising sharply (*see* Figure 16.1). During the first nine months that the clinic was open, these numbers remained stable and over the next year began to fall sharply and have not regained their former levels. The proportion of deaths involving methadone also fell and actual numbers of methadone-related deaths have remained stable at a very low level in spite of hugely increased amounts of methadone prescribed and dispensed in the city.[24,25] This supports previous evidence[26] that methadone treatment can prevent heroin deaths, whilst reinforcing the fact that methadone itself can be prescribed and dispensed safely.

Wider primary care

After one year, numbers of patients treated with methadone by GPs outside the clinic had approximately doubled. A local training programme was set up for GPs to gain informal advice and support about patients with drug-related problems. Meanwhile, a number of local GPs undertook the Royal College of GPs Certificate in the Management of Drug Misuse. The clinic regularly has GP registrars and medical students attached. In addition to this, various training sessions are regularly carried out by members of the clinic for other groups such as GP registrars, doctors specialising in psychiatry, and medical students.

Research evaluation

The clinic was the subject of a cohort study of the outcomes of methadone treatment in this setting.[21] Further groups of patients in the clinic became participants in studies of children of heroin users (funded by the European Commission), safer benzodiazepine prescribing (funded by the Drug Action Team) and arrest referrals (funded by the Home Office). In this way the almost unique opportunity of having a large number of previously untreated patients entering treatment was exploited to the full in terms of contributing to the evidence base.

Problems and solutions for service development

Dealing with hierarchies

Putting the initial idea for the clinic into action involved complex and prolonged negotiations between stakeholders. Sometimes this was due to political or administrative difficulties or lack of experience in dealing with large organisational hierarchies. Even after the clinic was running, difficulties were experienced with cumbersome NHS management procedures and remote structures. Personal contacts with dedicated individuals in each organisation who really wanted the project to succeed were the key to pushing things forward.

Funding

NHS funding is precariously constructed year on year according to shifting sets of government priorities and unpredictable overall funding, much of which is ring-fenced for specific purposes. After the initial stages of financial insecurity it was essential to establish a core budget from mainstream funding and, in order to do this, good relationships and joint working between the Drug Action Team, the PCT and the clinic had to be established and maintained. This was particularly important owing to the demise of health authorities following the restructuring of the NHS.

Liaison with other local organisations

Less opposition was encountered than anticipated. Local pharmacies co-operated enthusiastically as described above. Although the Local Medical Committee had initially expressed strong opposition to GPs working with heroin users, it ultimately welcomed and approved these developments.

The primary care service developed in a complementary way to the specialist service, with separate clinical governance structures. The development of clear protocols and agreed arrangements for joint working became a priority and continues in the context of overall service development in the city.

Continuing Development

Maintaining a 'primary care' identity

The clinic's perceived identity as a primary care-based service run by GPs has been essential in enabling its 'pump-priming' role to continue, and is central to the long-term harm minimisation ethos of the clinic. It has also contributed to the low cost of the service, in that ten-minute doctor appointments have been the mainstay, with patients accessing more intensive keyworking only at times of crisis. The development of the service has not discouraged local GPs from taking part in this work. The measurement of outcomes in terms of health improvements for patients and city-wide reduction in drug-related deaths has proved the key to demonstrating the success of the primary care approach.

Maintaining the philosophy of the clinic

The nature of harm minimisation is that it is a long-term palliative treatment for a chronic relapsing condition. Lack of 'cure' means a risk of political unpopularity and patients appearing to stagnate within the system. It may also appear that there is a 'bottomless pit' of unmet need. An important way of addressing this is to maintain a clear philosophy, remembering that the evidence base supports harm minimisation.

In short, the clinic aims to keep the patients alive and as healthy as possible until such time as they may be ready to become abstinent. The importance of this philosophy is that it faces the reality of heroin addiction without damaging morale by setting unrealistic goals.

Ongoing development

The clinic now offers the full range of community-based treatments for drug users. Proposed developments include satellites in outlying areas of the city and for drug users with particular needs, and enhanced links with other local services.

Conclusion

The Primary Care Clinic for Drug Dependence in Sheffield and the associated pharmacy scheme are now well established within the city. Central to success were the broad coalition of support for the service, clarity of goals, the fact that progress was measurable, and the carefully circumscribed area of work undertaken at least in the initial stages. This meant that local drug users and professionals could understand the clinic and its basis and how they might use it.

False hopes and expectations were not raised amongst drug users or the staff. Clear reliance on the existing evidence base for the clinic's protocol contributed to clarity of goals. It also meant that in a potentially risky field where patients have a high mortality and where professionals may be vulnerable, the clinic was able to treat patients within defined and defensible guidelines.

The development of the Primary Care Clinic for Drug Dependence has had a major impact on the care of drug users in the city and has allowed some hundreds of previously untreated drug users to access evidence-based treatment without any increase in treatment related deaths. The service is also highly cost effective. Whilst no one model of service can be appropriate for all localities, aspects of the Sheffield experience may prove helpful to communities and providers elsewhere.

References

1   Frischer M, Goldberg D and Green S (1993) How many drug injectors are there in the UK? *Int J Drug Policy*. 4: 190–3.

2   Healey A, Knapp M, Astin J, *et al.* (1998) Economic burden of drug dependency: social costs incurred by drug users at intake to the National Treatment Outcome Research Study. *Br J Psychiatry.* **173**: 160–5.

3   Kolar AF, Brown BS, Haertzen CA, *et al.* Children of substance abusers: the life experiences of children of opiate addicts in methadone maintenance. *Am J Drug Alcohol Abuse.* **20**: 159–71.

4   Ward J, Hall W and Mattick RP (1999) Role of maintenance treatment in opioid dependence. *Lancet.* **353**: 221–6.

5   Hutchinson S, Taylor A, Gruer L, *et al.* (2000) One year follow-up of opiate injectors treated with oral methadone in a GP-centred programme. *Addiction.* **95**(7): 1055–68.

6   Greenwood J (1990) Creating a new drug service in Edinburgh. *BMJ.* **300**: 587–9.

7   The Task Force to Review Services for Drug Misusers (1996) *Report of an Independent Review of Drug Treatment Services in England.* HMSO, London.

8   HMSO (1998) *Tackling Drugs to Build a Better Britain. The Government's 10 year strategy for tackling drug misuse.* HMSO, London.

9   Greenwood J (1992) Persuading general practitioners to prescribe: good husbandry or a recipe for chaos? *Br J Addict.* **87**: 567–74.

10   Glanz A (1986) Findings of a national survey of the role of general practitioners in the treatment of opiate misuse: views on treatment. *BMJ.* **293**: 543–5.

11   Merrill J and Ruben S (2000) Treating drug dependence in primary care: worthy ambition but flawed policy? *Drugs: Education, Prevention and Policy.* **7**(3): 203–12.

12   Department of Health (1999) *Drug Misuse and Dependence – guidelines on clinical management.* HMSO, London.

13   Robertson JR (1989) Treatment of drug misuse in the general practice setting. *Br J Addict.* **84**: 377–80.

14   Home Office (2000) Reducing Drug-related Deaths: a report by the advisery Council on the Misuse of Drugs. HMSO, London.

15   National Treatment Agency (2002) Models of Care for Treatment of Adult Drug Misusers. HMSO, London.

16   Marsch LA (1998) The efficacy of methadone maintenance interventions in reducing illicit opiate use, HIV risk behaviour and criminality: a meta-analysis. *Addiction.* **93**: 515–32.

17   Keen J, Rowse G, Mathers N, *et al.* (2000) Can methadone maintenance for heroin-dependent patients retained in general practice reduce criminal conviction rates and time spent in prison? *Br J Gen Pract.* **50**: 48–9.

18   Reno R and Aiken L (1993) Life activities and life quality of heroin addicts in and out of methadone treatment. *Int J Addict.* **28**(3): 211–32.

19   Magura S, Nwakeze PC and Demsky S (1998) Pre- and in treatment predictors of retention in methadone treatment using survival analysis. *Addiction.* **93**(1): 51–60.

20   Ball JC and Ross A (1991) *The Effectiveness of Methadone Maintenance Treatment.* Springer Verlag, New York.

21　Keen J, Oliver P, Rowse G and Mathers N (2003) Does methadone maintenance treatment based on the new national guidelines work in a primary care setting? *Br J Gen Practice*. (In press).

22　Gossop M, Marsden J, Stuart D, *et al.* (1999) Methadone treatment practices and outcomes for opiate addicts treated in drug clinics and in general practice: results from the Capital's National Treatment Outcome Research Study. *Br J Gen Pract*. **49**: 31–4.

23　Gossop M, Marsden J, Stewart D and Rolfe A (2000) Patterns of improvement after methadone treatment: 1 year follow-up results from the National Treatment Outcome Research Study (NTORS). *Drug Alcohol Depend*. **60**: 275–86.

24　Keen J, Oliver P and Mathers N (2002) Methadone maintenance treatment can be provided in a primary care setting without increasing methadone-related mortality: the Sheffield experience 1997–2000. *Br J Gen Pract*. **52**(478): 387–9.

25　Oliver P and Keen J (2003) Concomitant drugs of misuse and drug using behaviours associated with fatal opiate poisonings in Sheffield, England 1997–2000. *Addiction*. **98**: 191–7.

26　Gronbladh L, Ohland MS and Gunne L (1990) Mortality in heroin addiction: impact of methadone treatment. *Acta Psychiatrica Scandinivica*. **82**: 223–7.

CHAPTER 17

Engaging with the messy world of primary care and urban communities: future directions

Chris Drinkwater and Joe Kai

This book has explored a diversity of ways in which developing and delivering primary care in areas of urban disadvantage can be addressed. In this concluding chapter we attempt to draw together common themes and lessons. We relate these to critical challenges and opportunities for contemporary primary care, highlighted at the beginning of this volume and further here. We suggest how the creative approaches and solutions illustrated in this book might become part of the mainstream, and thus contribute to making a real difference to the health of people living in urban disadvantaged communities.

A value base

We started by looking at the personal stories of staff in a community health project and in a general practice (*see* Chapters 2 and 3). This was deliberate so that readers could feel, and perhaps identify with, the reality of inner city work, its stresses, and challenges, and its rewards. The two things that come across in both these chapters are the respect and trust for people within the communities that are served and the close and trusting working relationships that exist within these teams.

The next three chapters followed apparently contradictory themes.

Chapter 4 examined ways of addressing the public health needs of the whole community. Chapter 5 looked at the stresses and tensions faced by healthcare staff in demanding roles, while Chapter 6 looked at how marrying community development and primary care can be used to strengthen and empower geographical communities and diverse communities of interest. Put slightly differently, the three themes that these chapters pursue are:

- engaging the public, local communities and service users
- engaging front-line staff
- delivering the public health agenda.

These are recurring themes in many of the subsequent accounts in the book about what can be achieved in practice. Their common thread is a value base about building trust, respect and networks with service users and front-line staff as a prerequisite to delivering public health outputs and outcomes.

Engaging the public and service users

Chapter 7 told of a community development approach to building a partnership between a primary care organisation and the local communities which it serves – Community Action on Health in Newcastle. Community Action on Health has been an organic and incremental development, which has had to make sense and win support from local people. It has also had to be sensitive to local circumstances. When the three Newcastle PCGs merged to form a single PCT, there was a deliberate attempt to maintain Community Action on Health as an organisation which served three discrete areas which made sense to local people, rather than becoming a single central organisation. It will be interesting to see how long this can be sustained in the face of a national agenda about establishing a single patient forum (PF) in each PCT.

These PFs will be supported by an outreach team of workers who are employed by and accountable to a national body, the Commission for Public and Patient Involvement in Health (CPPIH),[1] unlike Community Action on Health where the workers are accountable to a local management committee, largely composed of local people. Although there is a commitment from CPPIH to build on local developments, it is hard to see how a top down and a bottom up model can co-exist, particularly when the PF has the statutory responsibility to represent the views of local communities to the PCT and can also elect one of their members to sit as non-executive director on the trust board.

Rules of engagement

Community Action on Health highlights a number of questions about the time and hard work required to engage with service users and the public. This hasn't always been successful because engagement has remained problematic in some areas where there is little collective community action. But by and large the project workers have avoided the twin dangers of speaking on behalf of the community, thus excluding community representatives, and of balancing the need to challenge the system with the need to work in co-operation with it.[2]

Their greatest challenge now is about maintaining the ethos and the values of the approach, while their aims and purpose become part of the mainstream. They have to decide whether to remain independent or to become part of a larger picture which will inevitably be more formal and will include statutory responsibilities which are likely to change the way the organisation operates.

The two subsequent chapters (8 and 9) look at engagement from the perspective of a parent involved in a Sure Start Programme and from the perspectives of young people in a disadvantaged area. Both clearly identify how involvement has led to improved confidence and self-belief, as well as the development of new skills, something that is not always acknowledged in an increasingly output and outcome led culture. Just as significantly, these accounts stress how important it is for staff to reflect and learn new ways of working, if they are to engage effectively with service users.

Engaging front-line staff

Overcoming the fix-it mentality

Donald Schon in *The Reflective Practitioner: how professionals think in action*[3] has highlighted the 'hard high ground of technical rationality' and the 'swamp' where problems are messy, confusing and incapable of technical solution. He also noted that the problems of greatest human concern are usually located in the swamp.

This analysis neatly encapsulates an enduring problem: the expert paternalistic model of professional practice and the current hierarchical power structures within the NHS, where acute and tertiary hospitals and doctors remain the dominant force (hard technical high ground), rather than primary care and the community (in the swamp). The service rationale is predominantly about fixing episodes of illness rather than developing relationships, continuity and support for people to take responsibility for their own health.

The consequence for professional behaviour is that we are often better at creating dependency than autonomy, with the inevitable corollary, that when things go wrong, we end up getting blamed. Another consequence of this fix-it mentality is that when things get tough we tend to retreat into our tribal networks where we, by and large, deal with the consequences of ill health, rather than taking a broad inter-agency and inter-professional approach to dealing with the causes of ill health.

Shifting the Balance of Power Within the NHS: securing delivery[4] states that:

'Staff need to be involved in decisions which affect service delivery. Empowerment comes when staff own the policies and are able to bring about real change.'

Hopefully, this now points in a new direction by making a clear and explicit link between empowering front-line staff and empowering the public and service users. The same engagement agenda applies to both groups and can only be delivered by developing more open, democratic and accountable structures.

Reflecting on the contributions to this book, there is a clear sense that one of the most effective mechanisms for engaging front-line staff is to support them in developing systematic approaches to patient and public involvement. Involvement in service development results in the development of services which are responsive to local need. It can also be responsible for changing the still too common paternalistic approaches of service providers to a more open and accountable culture in which professionals work in partnership with local communities and service providers.

Developing inter-professional working

The other drivers for change are a clear recognition of the need to break down tribal professional and inter-agency barriers and to move towards more collaborative inter-professional and inter-agency approaches. This, in common with local government initiatives to foster participatory democracy, has the potential to lead to better mechanisms for local accountability.

The implications are that health professionals will need to develop a new set of skills which are about horizontal rather than vertical (delegation downwards/accountability upwards) working. These new skills will have to include local networking, building mutuality of interests, facilitation and valuing diversity and joint working.

The major challenges to this agenda are the current crises in recruitment and retention across all professional groups, which are particularly marked in areas of social disadvantage, and the issues identified in Chapter 5, including:

'role overload, difficulties with superiors, role conflict (for example between family and work) and low participation and control in non-medical staff.'

There is an inherent danger in focusing on meeting recruitment and retention targets at the expense of addressing key issues about the role and nature of professional practice in the 21st century. Increasing the numbers without paying attention to the systems in which people work is unlikely to be successful.

Staff need to be offered the possibility of autonomy to develop locally accountable services within an agreed framework which provides flexibility and choice. The reality, if not the rhetoric, seems to be moving in the opposite direction, with the centre trying to maintain control through an increasing array of national targets, performance indicators and systems of inspection. The danger of this approach is that it runs the risk of creating dysfunctional organisations, which absorb energies and resources that could more productively be directed elsewhere. And as Jenny Firth-Cozens demonstrates in Chapter 5, dysfunctional organisations produce demoralised and demotivated staff.

Delivering the public health agenda in practice

In all the projects illustrated in this book, it is clear that what they are delivering is public health in practice. They are supporting and encouraging front-line staff to work in different ways, they are targeting inequalities in health through working with socially excluded groups and they are developing effective and sustainable local partnerships. This broad definition of public health does not always sit easily with a narrower specialist public health function that is focused on best practice, best value, evidence-based medicine and performance management.

The tension between a system that uses nationally set performance management targets as a means of central command and control, and a dispersed local model in which staff are given autonomy and choice within an agreed framework threatens to undermine real progress. The central control model is akin to a simple bio-medical system in which variables can be controlled and input of standardised resources will produce standardised outputs. The dispersed local model reflects a more complex social system in which locally sensitive ways of working have to be discovered because variables carry different weight and are impossible to control.

Not all that counts can be 'counted'

The current challenge for public health is to resist being overwhelmed by the siren voices of the hard technical high ground of evidence, formal needs assessment and centrally set targets. Instead it must engage with the messy world of primary care and community development where local context, partial evidence, uncertainty and vested interest dominate.

It is unlikely that a randomised controlled trial (RCT) will ever be designed that will effectively test whether or not building trust and relationships has a positive effect on health outcomes. In the same way it is difficult to see how an RCT could be used to assess any of the approaches described in this book. By their very nature these projects are about making connections and being broad and holistic. They do not focus down on a single clearly defined intervention and they do not have inclusion and exclusion criteria that help to identify the precise characteristics of individuals who might or might not benefit from the intervention.

Can public health return to its roots?

In some respects public health within PCTs has the opportunity to return to its Victorian roots. The introduction of improved sanitation, better housing and nutrition supported by partial evidence and often in the teeth of resistance from vested interests was well on the way to tackling deaths from infectious diseases long before the introduction of evidence-based antibiotics.[5] In the same way the projects in this book offer partial evidence and describe a way forward for tackling inequalities in mortality and morbidity due to our current epidemic of behavioural and chronic diseases. All will need the same sort of vision, commitment and energy, that the founders of public health demonstrated.

Mainstreaming new ways of working

Another common problem raised by all of these innovative projects is sustainability. Research into Collaboration and Co-ordination in Area-Based Initiatives (CCABI)[6] found three types of mainstreaming.

- Mainstreaming projects – the securing of funding to continue particular activities.
- Mainstreaming good practice – ensuring that a mainstream agency adapts and reproduces examples of good practice from initiative activity.
- Mainstreaming policy issues – when the policy lessons from the work have a direct influence on the policy process.

To an extent all of the projects discussed in this book have, at least initially, had to grapple with the issue of securing funding for particular approaches or activities but they have also been, to varying degrees, successful in mainstreaming the good practice that they have developed and in influencing the local policy agenda.

The meaning of mainstreaming

There is however another more restrictive view of mainstreaming which sees project activity as useful, only in as much as it delivers statutory sector targets. The problem with this approach is that it runs counter to the original meaning of the term. Mainstreaming originated in European Union policy on gender.[7] It indicates a process of ensuring the wider consideration of (and action on) issues that might otherwise be compartmentalised and disregarded by those specialising in a particular area of activity. For example, the position of women in engineering could be seen as an equality issue to be dealt with by agencies specialising in equality issues through dedicated funds, rather than to do with the way training is provided or factories run and so on.

The effect of mainstreaming is thus to challenge assumptions that any one sector, agency or profession is the repository of all knowledge, and in doing so to place a particular emphasis on partnerships. As a result, the benefits can go in all directions – not just to the dominant force in any particular sphere of activity.

Occupying a new middle ground

The danger of a restrictive view of mainstreaming has been identified by a recent report called *Inside Out: rethinking inclusive communities*.[8] This surveyed over 40 community-based projects and confirmed that they are a vital link to socially excluded communities because they have developed trust by filling the gaps between mainstream services. However, concerns were also expressed that where such organisations acted as 'instruments of government policy', they risked compromising their independence and losing the trust of the people they serve.

The three principles that this report proposes for developing inclusive communities resonate with many of those within the projects described in this book, namely:

- service innovation and learning which focus on people-based solutions
- trusting community-based organisations, which in turn allows them to win the trust of the people they serve
- creating a 'new middle ground' to enable community power-sharing and avoiding organisation mismatches.

The challenge for all of the projects for mainstreaming is to ensure that they continue to occupy this middle ground. Here they can mediate between the needs of the people and communities that they serve and the bureaucratic and hierarchical structures of the statutory agencies.

Reflective learning

As we discuss in Chapter 1, adopting principles and approaches to develop learning organisations can enable and sustain progress. The framework outlined in Box 17.1 is partly based on what has and has not worked for the projects and approaches this book has illustrated, and partly based on useful guidance for developing a health programme as part of neighbourhood renewal.[9]

Box 17.1: Developing reflective learning

Step 1: Be clear about the issue that you want to address
- Identify and gather any baseline information that may be available about this issue.
- What initiatives and services are currently in place to address this issue?
- Are the current programmes effective?
- What is the importance of this issue for national, regional and local priorities?

Step 2: Engage with all of the key people and groups who have an interest in the issue
- Find out the views of existing service users and of local people and community groups.
- Ensure the right people are involved in the discussion, including those who may be opposed to or feel threatened by any change.

- Listen and respond to any issues or concerns that are raised and think through what compromises may or may not be acceptable.

Step 3: Develop and test out your programme or intervention
- What is known about the issue, in terms of best practice and what works elsewhere?
- Be clear about the vision, values and purpose of the initiative.
- Clarify and make explicit the approach to be used and the processes and pathways that will be followed.
- Identify potential outputs and outcomes, including intermediate process outcomes.
- Recruit staff that have the personal skills and competencies to deliver the programme.

Step 4: Programme delivery and maintenance
- Ensure that early monitoring and review are built into the programme, including feedback from service users.
- Ensure that there are regular meetings of the project team and of key partners so that ownership and involvement in the project are maintained and the values and philosophy of the project are re-affirmed.
- Be prepared to adapt or change the project in response to feedback or changing local needs. Learn from mistakes and difficulties.
- For single worker projects ensure that there are good support mechanisms in place.

Step 5: Sustainability and mainstreaming
- Take every opportunity to market the outcomes of the project to funders and key policy makers.
- Ensure that you submit reports to funders and accountable bodies on time and in the appropriate format.
- Build trust and alliances with front-line staff, service users and the local community so that they are in a position to support and advocate the project.
- Demonstrate how the project is helping statutory agencies to meet delivery targets.
- Think through the issues of mainstreaming. Is the main aim to sustain the project as it is or to disseminate and spread the good practice and to influence policy makers? Or is it to do a combination of these?
- Retain innovative and flexible approaches and be alert to policy changes and new funding opportunities.

Getting real about new approaches

Devising new policies and agreeing strategies are easy. Doing more needs assessment and research is easy. Operationalising new approaches that deliver change and better outcomes in partnership with service users, local people and local communities is not. As the accounts in this book recognise, it is hard, challenging work. It means having the courage to get off the hard ground and move into the swamp, to engage with the complex, the human and the social world. But, when it is successful, it is immensely rewarding. More time and effort need to be devoted to supporting the leadership, skills and competencies required to do this sort of work. Returning to where we started in our introduction to this book, the opportunities and benefits of linking social capital, empowerment and health can then be realised more frequently and with more force. As the accounts in this book have demonstrated, this requires vision and commitment together with the development of relationships of trust and respect for service users and local people.

References

1   Department of Health (2002) *Involving Patients and the Public in Healthcare: response to the listening exercise*. DoH, London.

2   Crowley P, Green J, Freake D and Drinkwater C (2002) Primary Care Trusts involving the community: is community development the way forward? *J Manage Med.* **16**(4); 311–22.

3   Schon D (1983) *The Reflective Practitioner: how professionals think in action*. Temple Smith, London.

4   Department of Health (2001) *Shifting the Balance of Power within the NHS: securing delivery*. DoH, London.

5   McKeown T (1976) *The Role of Medicine: dream, mirage or nemesis*. Nuffield Provincial Hospitals Trust, London.

6   Department of Employment (2000) *Collaboration and Co-ordination in Area-Based Initiatives*. DoE, Transport and the Regions, London.

7   Rubery J (2002) Gender Mainstreaming and Equality in the EU. *Industrial Relations Journal* **33**: 500–22.

8   Barrow Cadbury Trust (2003) *Inside out: rethinking inclusive communities*. A Demos Report supported by the Barrow Cadbury Trust. www.demos.co.uk

9   Department of Health/Neighbourhood Renewal Unit (2002) *Health and Neighbourhood Renewal: Guidance from the Department of Health and the Neighbourhood Renewal Unit*. DoH/NRV, London.

Index